Mobile Wearable Nano-Bio Health Monitoring Systems with Smartphones as Base Stations

Vijay K. Varadan and
Linfeng Chen

Co-published by Momentum Press, LLC, 222 E. 46th Street, #203, New York, NY 10017, USA (www.momentumpress.net)

A catalog record is available from the Library of Congress.

Print ISBN: 978-1-60650-424-6

Electronic ISBN: 978-1-60650-414-7

Series Editors' Preface

Biomedical and Nanomedical Technologies (B&NT)
This **concise** monograph series focuses on the implementation of various engineering principles in the conception, design, development, analysis and operation of biomedical, biotechnological and nanotechnology systems and applications. The primary objective of the series is to compile the latest research topics in biomedical and nanomedical technologies, specifically devices and materials.

Each volume comprises a collection of invited manuscripts, written in an accessible manner and of a concise and manageable length. These timely collections will provide an invaluable resource for initial enquiries about technologies, encapsulating the latest developments and applications with reference sources for further detailed information. The content and format have been specifically designed to stimulate further advances and applications of these technologies by reaching out to the non-specialist across a broad audience.

Contributions to *Biomedical and Nanomedical Technologies* will inspire interest in further research and development using these technologies and encourage other potential applications. This will foster the advancement of biomedical and nanomedical applications, ultimately improving healthcare delivery.

Editor:
Ahmed Al-Jumaily, PhD, Professor of Biomechanical Engineering & Director of the Institute of Biomedical Technologies, Auckland University of Technology.

Associate Editors:
Waqar Ahmed, PhD, Chair, Nanotechnology and Advanced Manufacturing, and Head, Institute of Nanotechnology and Bioengineering, School of Computing, Engineering & Physical Sciences, University of Central Lancashire, UK.

Christopher H.M. Jenkins, PhD, PE, Professor and Head, Mechanical & Industrial Engineering Department, Montana State University.

Preface

Due to the rapid advances in nanotechnology, telecommunication and information technologies, efficient and reliable telemedicine (also known as remote point of care or remote healthcare), which has been a holy grail in medicine, is coming into practice. It is expected to significantly improve the quality of healthcare while reducing the costs, especially for patients with chronic illnesses, such as neurological, metabolic, and cardiovascular disorders which require constant long term untethered monitoring, as well as patients discharged after an operation or serious medical crises. It eliminates the distance barriers in medicine. Vital information about a patient, who lives far away from medical support, can be acquired by the medical staff. More importantly it saves lives in critical care and emergency situations by alerting medical staff if there is a dangerous change in patient status.

This monograph discusses the development and application of mobile wearable nano-bio health monitoring systems for telemedicine. In such a system, nanomaterials-based biosensors are used to measure physiological signals, such as electrocardiogram (ECG), electroencephalogram (EEG), electromyogram (EMG), and electrooculogram (EOG). The obtained physiological signals are filtered, amplified and transmitted to a remote storage server, utilizing Smartphones as base stations. Cloud computing resources are used for complex computations, such as feature extraction and automatic diagnosis. The information in the remote storage server can be instantly accessed by healthcare providers, and medical advice can also be sent instantly to the patient through the wireless communication system.

This monograph consists of six chapters. The first chapter starts with the evolution of health monitoring. The basic architecture of a mobile health monitoring system is discussed subsequently, followed by the applications of Smartphones for healthcare. Following this, smart textile based wearable health monitoring systems are discussed.

Chapters 2 and 3 discuss the technologies for the development of mobile wearable nano-bio health monitoring systems. Chapter 2 deals with the development of nano-bio sensors for health monitoring, which exhibit attractive advantages over the conventional physiological sensors. After introducing the typical physiological signals for health monitoring, bioelectric sensors based on carbon nanotubes and metal nanowires, respectively, are discussed, followed by cuffless blood pressure sensors. Chapter 3 discusses the telecommunication and information technologies for mobile health monitoring systems, and the discussion is concentrated on signal transmission and receiving, and the relaying of signals by Smartphones. Following this, e-Nanoflex is discussed as an example of the telecommunication and data processing system.

Chapter 4 discusses the development of smart textile based wearable health monitoring systems. After introducing the concept of smart textiles, printable electronics are discussed, followed by textile sensor technology. Subsequently, the roll-to-roll techniques for the fabrication of smart-textile based health monitoring systems are discussed.

Four case studies are given in Chapter 5. These are cardiac health monitoring, e-bra for ECG measurement for women, smart vest for ECG and blood pressure measurement for men, and diagnosis of sleep apnea.

In Chapter 6, a brief summary is made on the transformation of healthcare practices due to mobile wearable health monitoring systems, and the technical challenges for the development and application of mobile wearable health monitoring systems are discussed.

The development of mobile wearable health monitoring systems for telemedicine is an interdisciplinary field, mainly involving nanotechnology, electrical and electronic engineering, information technology, biology and medicine. The authors have many years of research experience in this field. This monograph is prepared mainly based on the authors' research results, and some of the technical details are released for the first time. Meanwhile, the major achievements and the latest progress in this area are reviewed in the monograph.

The authors greatly appreciate the contributions from Pratyush Rai, Prashanth Kumar, Sechang Oh, Hyeokjun Kwon and Nilanjan Banerjee. These people spent a lot of time and effort in the design and implementation of various types of mobile wearable health monitoring systems, and their careful comments greatly improved the contents of this monograph.

This monograph can be a textbook for a short training course on telemedicine, as well as a reference for nanotechnology courses for graduates and senior undergraduates in the fields of electrical and electronic engineering, materials sciences and engineering, physics, chemistry, biology, and medicine. Engineers and healthcare practitioners who are interested in telemedicine will also find this monograph a useful reference.

Author Biographies

Vijay K. Varadan is currently the Twenty-First Century Endowed Chair in Nano-and Bio-Technology and Medicine, and Distinguished Professor of Electrical Engineering and Distinguished Professor of Biomedical Engineering (College of Engineering) and Neurosurgery (College of Medicine) at University of Arkansas. He is also a Professor of Neurosurgery at the Pennsylvania State University College of Medicine. He also holds honorary doctorate degrees in Nano-, and Bio-Technologies and Medicine from India. He joined the University of Arkansas in January 2005 after serving on the faculty of Cornell University, Ohio State University and Pennsylvania State University for the past 39 years. He is also the Director of the Center of Excellence for Nano-, Micro-, and Neuro-Electronics, Sensors and Systems and the Director of the NSF Center for Wireless Nanosensors and Systems (WiNS). He is also a Director of the Global Institute of Nanotechnology in Engineering and Medicine (GINTEM). The purpose of this Institute is to create a global effort to solve current and future medical concerns using advanced nanotechnologies by developing Research Hospitals at selected overseas countries. Varadan has concentrated on the design and development of various electronic, acoustic and structural composites, smart materials, structures, and devices including sensors, transducers, Microelectromechanical Systems (MEMS), synthesis and large scale fabrication of carbon nanotubes, NanoElectroMechanical Systems (NEMS), microwave, acoustic and ultrasonic wave absorbers and filters. He has developed neurostimulator, wireless microsensors and systems for sensing and control of Parkinson's disease, epilepsy, glucose in the blood and Alzheimer's disease. He is also developing both silicon and organic based wireless sensor systems with RFID for human gait analysis and sleep disorders and various neurological disorders. He was a founder and the Editor-in-Chief of the Journal of Smart Materials and Structures. He was the founder and Editor-in-Chief of the Journal of Nanotechnology in Engineering and Medicine. He is currently the Editor-in-Chief of the Journal of Smart Nanosystems in Engineering and Medicine, and Editor of the Journal of Advanced Materials Research. He is an Associate Editor of the Journal of Microlithography, Microfabrication and Microsystem. He serves on the editorial board of International Journal of Computational Methods. He has published more than 500 journal papers and 15 books. He has 15 patents pertinent to conducting polymers, smart structures, smart antennas, phase shifters, carbon nanotubes, and implantable device for Parkinson's patients, MEMS accelerometers and gyroscopes. He is a fellow of SPIE, ASME, Institute of Physics, Acoustical Society of America. He has many visiting professorship appointments in leading schools overseas.

Linfeng Chen received his B. Sc. degree in modern applied physics (major) and his B.Eng. degree in machine design and manufacture (minor) from the Tsinghua University, Beijing, China, in 1991, and he received his PhD. degree in physics from the National University of Singapore in 2001. From 1991 to 1994, he was an assistant lecturer at the Department of Modern Applied Physics, Tsinghua University, Beijing, China. From 1994 to 1997, he was a research scholar with the Department of Physics, National University of Singapore. From 1997 to 2001, he worked at the DSO National Laboratories, Singapore, as a project engineer and later a member of technical staff. From 2001 to 2005, he was a research scientist at the Temasek Laboratories, National University of Singapore. Since 2005, he has been a member of research faculty at the Department of Electrical Engineering, University of Arkansas, Fayetteville. He is a senior member of IEEE. His research interests mainly include microwave electronics, functional nanomaterials, and energy harvesting and storage devices.

Contents

Abstract

This monograph discusses the development and application of mobile wearable nano-bio health monitoring systems for telemedicine. In such a system, nanomaterials-based biosensors are used to measure physiological signals, such as electrocardiogram (ECG), electroencephalogram (EEG), electromyogram (EMG), and electrooculogram (EOG). The obtained physiological signals are filtered, amplified and transmitted to a remote storage server, utilizing Smartphones as base stations. Cloud computing resources are used for complex computations, such as feature extraction and automatic diagnosis. The information in the remote storage server can be instantly accessed by healthcare providers, and medical advice can also be sent instantly to the patient through the wireless communication system.

1. Introduction

1.1 Evolution of health monitoring

Continuous health monitoring is essential for recuperating patients and patients with chronic health conditions. It can be used in judging whether an individual is in a physiological state suitable for his duties, and it is also useful for people of all age groups who have possible health problems or have opted for a healthy lifestyle.

Chronic diseases can be effectively controlled if they are diagnosed at their early stages and they are regularly monitored with proper medication cares and guides [1]. For example, detection of cardiac arrhythmias from continuous electrocardiogram (ECG) recordings is an important approach that physicians use to adjust medication for post myocardial infarction patients. Common chronic neurological disorders, such as epilepsy and Alzheimer's disease, can be identified from electroencephalogram (EEG) recordings. The changes in brain function may occur several hours before any clinical manifestation in patients with progressive brain ischemia, or in patients suffering from vasospasms after a subarachnoid hemorrhage. These events are important parts of a patient's health history, and the detection and recording of these events play a key role in the risk stratification process used by physicians to plan treatments. Therefore, continuous real time monitoring is a valuable tool that can help both diagnosis and treatment planning.

Many accidents, which have frequently happened on aircraft, high-speed passenger trains, long-range highway express buses and so on, were caused by the operational errors of the pilots or drivers [2]. Most of the operational errors were due to the high mental stress or drive dozing of the pilots or drivers, and some of them were diagnosed as sleep apnea syndrome (SAS). Diseases such as SAS and sudden infant death syndrome (SIDS) mostly happen while an individual is in sleep or in an unconscious condition. These diseases are generally difficult to detect by physicians without a continuous monitoring of the change in a person's vital signs. Therefore, close and continuous monitoring is needed, which can assist healthcare providers to identify whether a patient is in a healthy condition.

The concept of continuous health monitoring can be translated as point-of-care (POC) technology for preventive/corrective medicine, and as metabolic rate estimation and regulation in healthy lifestyle. POC testing is also known as ancillary testing, near-patient testing, and bedside testing. A classical definition of POC testing is "diagnostic testing performed at or near the site of patient care", and it is also defined as "analytical patient testing activity provided within the institution but performed outside the physical facilities of the clinical laboratories" [3].

A currently available system for POC monitoring consists of wired sensors which need to be manually mounted on a patient. Such a system has three obvious drawbacks. First, complete health monitoring needs multiple sensors to detect various physiological signals, such as ECG, EEG, electromyogram (EMG), electroculogram (EOG), pulse oximetry, air flow pressure, and respiration effort, and wiring these sensors to one monitoring unit is cumbersome and highly intrusive. Second, these sensors use customized data transmission hardware and software that cannot be easily integrated into a patient's quotidian life, and the individual has to carry a special device for data collection. Third, the sensors used in a majority of these systems are not wearable.

A conventional POC testing usually requires the transportation of instruments to the patient's premises for data collection at certain regular intervals. This traditional approach to POC systems usually involves frequent visits by healthcare personnel to the patient's vicinity for diagnosis. During these visits, the healthcare personnel usually record the patient's vital signs and take decisions as to any changes in the treatment and address any issues that the patient may have. Obviously this involves large expense in addition to the inconvenience caused to the patient in terms of the time spent and the intervention with daily life.

A higher quality of life is now expected by patients, even when suffering from various chronic diseases. Patients generally want to be treated at home and with as little pain and discomfort as possible. Society needs to reduce the increasing cost of medicine while also improving the quality of healthcare [4]. This implies a development of alternative solutions to the traditional hospital methods for disease prevention and health monitoring. Cost-efficient access to the best care and illness prevention can empower each individual and enable him/her to have a longer and healthier life.

Remote patient monitoring (RPM) is an emerging area of telemedicine, which includes devices and technology that enable healthcare providers to remotely diagnose, treat, and advise patients. RPM systems usually monitor a patient's vital signs, which could include ECG, EEG, respiration rate, blood pressure and temperature, depending upon the condition to be monitored. Such a system can obviate the need for repeated visits to the hospital. Moreover, the continuously monitoring of human physiology by such a system can provide valuable data to prognosticate the onset of critical health problems.

Recently, the concept of body area network (BAN) was proposed [5]. It is defined as a network of independent wireless nodes that span the personal space of a user. As an ultimate objective of BAN, the independent sensors for physiological signals, such as ECG, EOG, EMG, pulse rate, blood oxygen saturation, temperature and respiration, will send data through their wireless transmitters, to a single receiving station which may be a Smartphone, a personal digital assistant (PDA), a personal computer (PC), or a custom receiver unit. Various wireless communication protocols can be used, such as Bluetooth, ZigBee, and custom communication protocols for low power transmission of data.

A mobile wearable health monitoring system is a truest embodiment of the BAN concept [6]. Its body worn sensors (slaves) communicate with a single receiver unit (master) and transmit time synchronized data in real time. Mobile wearable health monitoring systems represent a new generation of healthcare by providing real-time unobtrusive health monitoring through the on-body sensors [7, 8].

Besides monitoring physiological parameters [9], a wearable health monitoring system can also be designed for monitoring body motions [6, 10–12]. The monitoring of human movement is important for the clinical applications of fall detection, fall risk assessment, and energy expenditure. The importance of these applications is considerable in light of the global demographic trends and the resultant rise in the occurrence of injurious falls and the decrease of physical activity [6]. The use of wearable motion sensing technology offers important advantages over conventional methods for obtaining measures of physical activity and/or physical functioning in individuals with chronic diseases. Having the capability to track human body kinematics allows clinicians to classify and analyze a stroke patient's progress which aid in the rehabilitation program. Monitoring and capturing real time body motion further permits corrective measures to be implemented for more effective rehabilitation results [11].

A considerable amount of research has been made on mobile wearable health monitoring systems, and encouraging progress has been achieved. This monograph aims to report the latest advances in the development of mobile wearable nano-bio health monitoring systems, and more information on in this field can be found in books [13, 14], reviews [10, 15–17], and numerous papers and presentations.

1.2 Architecture of a mobile health monitoring system

In this section, the e-Nanoflex platform developed by Varadan et al. [18] is used as an example for discussing the basic architecture of a mobile wearable health monitoring system. This platform is capable of monitoring the health condition of a patient wherever he/she may be and communicating the data in real time to a physician or a hospital. Unlike the conventional health monitoring systems that either are local sensor systems or rely on custom relaying devices, e-Nanoflex is a highly nonintrusive and inexpensive end-to-end cyber-physical system. Using nanostructured sensors, e-Nanoflex provides nearly invisible monitoring of physiological conditions. It relies on Smartphones to filter, compress, and relay geo-tagged data. Further, it ties to a backend cloud infrastructure for data storage, data dissemination, and abnormality detection using machine learning techniques. An e-Nanoflex is a complete system for physiological sensing and geo-tagged data dissemination to hospitals and caregivers. It is a basic platform that can support any nanostructure based flexible sensors for monitoring a variety of conditions such as body temperature, respiration air flow, oxygen consumption, bioelectric signals, pulse oximetry, muscle activity, and neural activity.

Advances in medical nanotechnology coupled with rapid development in Smartphones and cloud computing offer significant advantages over existing systems. Nanosensors offer the unique advantage of small size and high sensitivity that makes them ideally suited for everyday use as they bear no conspicuous presence. Additionally, a Smartphone can be used to relay health and activity monitoring data from these user worn devices to a cloud resident server. As shown in Figure 1-1, an e-Nanoflex system can seamlessly integrate nanobiosensors with Smartphone relays and backend cloud services to provide continuous health monitoring to patients.

As a basic platform, an e-Nanoflex can support a variety of sensors, such as nanostructure based flexible gas sensors, as well as carbon nanotube (CNT) based flexible strain and temperature sensors. Figure 1-2 shows an application example of an e-Nanoflex for monitoring respiration effort using a sensor incorporated in a band aid, which will be discussed further in Section 3.5. Other physiological signals, such as EOG, EEG, ECG and pulse rate, can also be monitored when corresponding sensors are used. More application examples can be found in the case studies discussed in Chapter 5.

An e-Nanoflex sensor system integrates a Bluetooth radio module, amplifier, and sensor in a compact medical plaster form. The system is easy to use and the sensors can be simply placed on the skin at appropriate positions, such as the limb lead positions for ECG. The data from the sensors are streamed to a backend cloud through a Smartphone. While initial

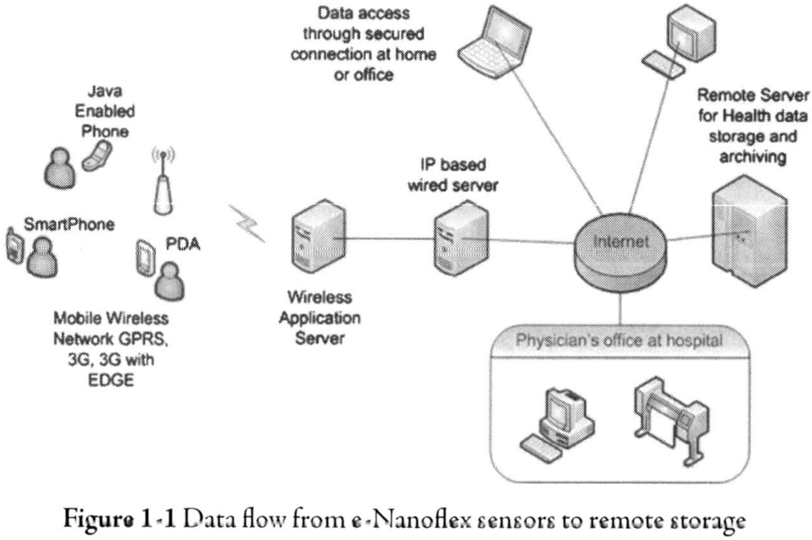

Figure 1-1 Data flow from e-Nanoflex sensors to remote storage servers.

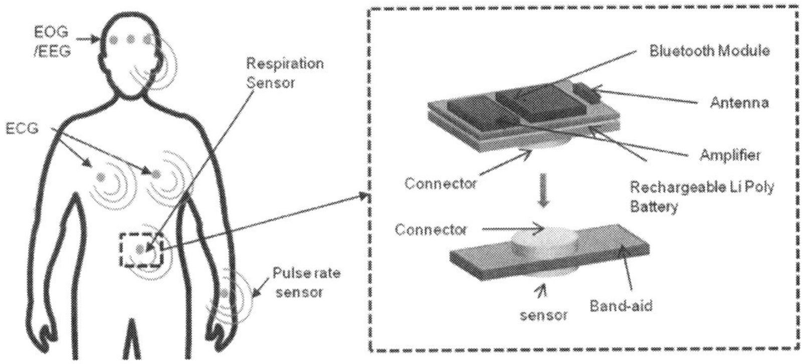

Figure 1-2 Monitoring of respiration effort using a sensor incorporated in a band aid.

filtering occurs locally at the Smartphone, most of the complex processing is delegated to the cloud. Such a partitioning approach has a two-fold advantage. First, sophisticated computationally intensive signal conditioning algorithms, such as adaptive filters, are best implemented on a server capable of cloud computing. Second, in anticipation of a large scale deployment, there will be multiple users sending data simultaneously and cloud storage is indispensable to handle such large volumes of data. Additionally, an alert message to a physician's phone or a message to the nearest emergency response service can be sent if any anomaly is detected by the cloud server. The Smartphone can also be programmed to automatically capture a video during a cardiac episode so that paramedics can be better prepared.

The data from the e-Nanoflex sensors can be displayed on the Smartphone, as shown in Figure 1-3 (a), so that the user can check the status

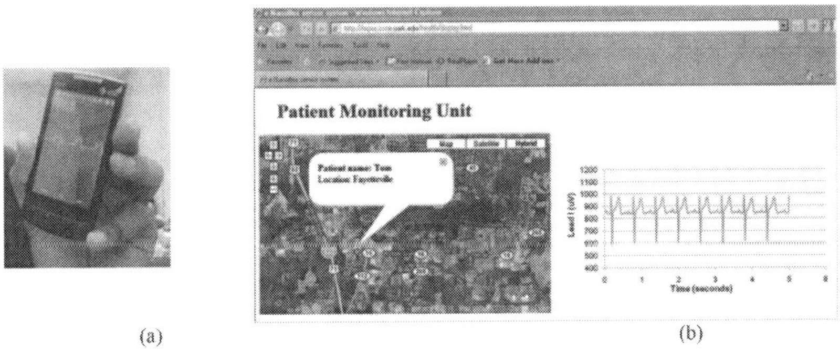

Figure 1-3 The data display, storage and recovery in an e-Nanoflex system. (a) A Smartphone displaying ECG data. (b) Snapshot of ECG data stored from a user and the corresponding location from which the data were sent.

anytime. The data, tagged with the current GPS location and the time, are also sent to a remote server through the 3G network. In case of an emergency, a message with recorded data and current location and time can be sent to the emergency response team. As shown in Figure 1-3 (b), the location of the user and the data received from the sensor can be recovered from the server.

1.3 Smartphones for healthcare applications

In the e-Nanoflex platform discussed in Section 1.2, a Smartphone not only works as a base station, but also performs basic analysis on the raw data from the sensors.

Smartphones are mobile telephones that have computer-like functionality, which typically includes e-mail, Internet access, and increasingly, some sort of screen and keyboard that allow use of software designed for Smartphones [19]. They are actually minicomputers that have a telephone attached. The first Smartphone was the Simon, designed by IBM in 1992. The real start of the Smartphone, in terms of public exposure, occurred in 2001 with the Palm "Treo", which had a full keyboard, wireless Web browsing, e-mail, calendar, and the ability to be synced with a computer to download third-party programs. In 2007, Apple released the iPhone, which had two primary innovations [19]. First, it used a touchscreen interface instead of a keyboard. The second significant innovation was not the device itself, but the App Store, a place where iPhone users could buy software designed specifically for the iPhone. Apple also opened the App Store to third-party designers and made a very low entry point, so small developers could participate.

Since Apple announced their mobile App Store in 2009, thousands of apps for the iPhone related to health or medicine have been developed [19]. The medically related Smartphone apps are not exclusive to the iPhone. Many companies that have developed medical applications for Smartphones are making them compatible for other brands as well, including Palm, Blackberry, Win Mobile, and Android.

Many healthcare providers are adopting Smartphones successfully in a diverse range of practices [19]. Several reasons make Smartphones attractive to healthcare providers. The primary reason is that many POC Smartphone apps have been developed. The second reason is that healthcare providers are mobile workers and a Smartphone provides a huge amount of information at their fingertips no matter where they are. Even when a healthcare provider is in his office, he is moving around a lot, not really stationed at his computer. Further, the multiple media aspects of Smartphones, along with connectivity and mobility can help a healthcare provider become more efficient. Meanwhile, patients are also getting used to accessing health information, actively participating in their own healthcare, and maintaining contact with their healthcare providers through Smartphones. In particular, chronic conditions such as diabetes, mellitus and cardiovascular disease, are perceived as a special niche market for Smartphone apps. Therefore, Smartphones are starting a new epoch in healthcare, and there are significant opportunities to exploit the potential of Smartphones in healthcare [20].

1.4 Smart textile based wearable health monitoring systems

Due to the advances in nanotechnologies, telecommunication, low-power design, new textiles, and flexible sensors, new user-friendly devices have been developed to enhance the comfort and security of a patient. As clothes and textiles are in direct contact with about ninety percent of the skin surface, smart sensors and smart clothes with noninvasive sensors are an attractive solution for home-based and ambulatory health monitoring [4].

Although it started off as an effort to address battlefield needs, the creation of a wearable information infrastructure, in the form of a smart shirt, opened up entirely new frontiers in civilian healthcare, including monitoring of firefighters at a fire scene, patients in hospitals or at home recovering from illnesses/surgeries, infants prone to cot death or sudden infant death syndrome (SIDS), or athletes in training or competition [21].

The field of smart textile-based wearable healthcare monitoring systems has been generating a lot of interest in the research and business communities, with the aim of getting the technology into the marketplace [2, 22]. For example, Coyle et al. developed a wearable sensing system that integrates a textile-based fluid handling system for sample collection and transport with a number of sensors including the sensors for sweat rate, ECG, respiration, and blood oxygenation [23]. It can be used to monitor a number of physiological parameters together with sweat composition in real time. This has huge implications for the field of sports and human performance and opens a new field of research in the clinical setting.

Smart textile based wearable health monitoring systems can greatly enhance home healthcare and disease prevention [4]. For healthy subjects, the system will not only help the user to adopt a healthier lifestyle, but will also effectively improve personal performances due to better fitness and more effective ways of coping with stress. For individuals at risk of diseases, the system will provide adequate information on how to deal with individual risk factors like hypertension, obesity, diabetes, physical inactivity, and stress through personalized training plans. Early detection through long-term trend analysis will dramatically reduce the potential damages of severe events. For post-event patients, this system can significantly improve the rehabilitation process, and can detect possible complications at their early stages. Daily monitoring will enable new forms of personalized drug treatment and the self-administration of drug medication, according to the specific behaviors and circumstances of each individual. For chronic patients, intelligent biomedical clothes empower the user to better understand and self-manage the disease state. Early detection by continuous long-term monitoring is helpful for avoiding the occurrence of acute events and complications that may lead to hospitalization and extended hospital treatments.

This monograph consists of six chapters. After the introductory chapter, Chapter 2 discusses nanotechnology-based biosensors for health monitoring, and Chapter 3 discusses the telecommunication and information technologies for mobile health monitoring systems. Chapter 4 discusses the development of smart textile based wearable health monitoring systems. Four case studies are given in Chapter 5. In Chapter 6, perspectives and major technical challenges in the development and application of mobile wearable health monitoring systems are discussed.

2. Nano-bio sensors for health monitoring

This chapter discusses the development of nanotechnology based biomedical sensors that will be integrated into mobile wearable health monitoring systems. After introducing the physiological signals often used for health monitoring, three types of biomedical sensors are discussed, including bioelectric sensors based on carbon nanotubes, bioelectric sensors based on metal nanowires, and cuffless blood pressure sensors.

2.1 Physiological signals for health monitoring

The physiological signals for health monitoring generally fall into two categories: bioelectric signals such as ECG and EEG, and nonelectric biossignals such as arterial pulse wave, pulse rate and pulse transit time.

2.1.1 Electrocardiogram (ECG)

The electrocardiogram (ECG, or EKG from the German Elektrokardiogramm) is a noninvasive diagnostic test for observing the abnormalities in cardiac electrophysiology. It is a transthoracic interpretation of the electrical activity of the heart over a period of time, as detected by the electrodes attached to the outer surface of the skin. ECG monitoring is an efficient and important clinical technique in healthcare as information from an ECG test can be used to discover heart diseases, determine the rate and regularity of heart beats as well as the size and position of chambers, and also to evaluate the effects of drugs or specialized devices used to regulate the heart, such as a pacemaker [1].

The ECG signals come from the tiny electrical changes on the skin, which are caused when the heart muscle depolarizes during a heartbeat. At rest, each heart muscle cell has a negative charge across its cell membrane. Decreasing this negative charge towards zero, via the influx of the positive cations (Na^+ and Ca^{2+}) is called depolarization, which activates the mechanisms in the cell that cause it to contract. During each heartbeat, a healthy heart will have an orderly progression of a wave of depolarization that is triggered by the cells in the sinoatrial node, spreads out through the atrium, passes through the atrioventracular node and then spreads all over the ventricles. This procedure can be detected as tiny rises and falls in the voltage between two electrodes placed at the two sides of the heart, and displayed as a wavy line either on a screen or on a paper. This wavy line indicates the overall rhythm of the heart and the weaknesses in different parts of the heart muscles [24].

To obtain more information about heart activities, usually more than two electrodes are used, and they can be combined into a number of pairs. For example: left arm (LA), right arm (RA) and left leg (LL) electrodes form the three pairs LA+RA, LA+LL, and RA+LL. The output from each pair is called a lead. Each lead looks at the heart from a particular angle. Different types of ECGs can be referred to by the number of leads that are recorded, for example

3-lead, 5-lead or 12-lead ECGs. As shown in Figure 2-1 (a), a traditional 12-lead ECG system usually requires ten electrodes that are strategically placed on the chest and the extremities. In a 12-lead ECG system, twelve different electrical signals are recorded at approximately the same time, but this configuration is not practical for ambulatory patients. The continuous monitoring of all the 12-lead ECG signals is only required for high risk patients who have already been diagnosed with cardiovascular diseases (CVDs). Moreover, the use of a full 12-lead ECG system for everyday monitoring can be inconvenient and cumbersome. An alternative five electrode system that gives most of the diagnostic information that can be obtained by a 12-lead ECG system can be used for continuous monitoring instead [25]. As shown in Figure 2-1 (c), in a 5-lead ECG system, four electrodes are attached to the patient's torso (modified extremities), and the last electrode acts as the precordial or "V" electrode.

Figure 2-1 (b) shows the electrode positions for a 3-lead ECG system. All the three electrodes are attached to the patient's torso (modified extremity leads), and they are right arm (RA), left arm (LA) and left leg (LL). The

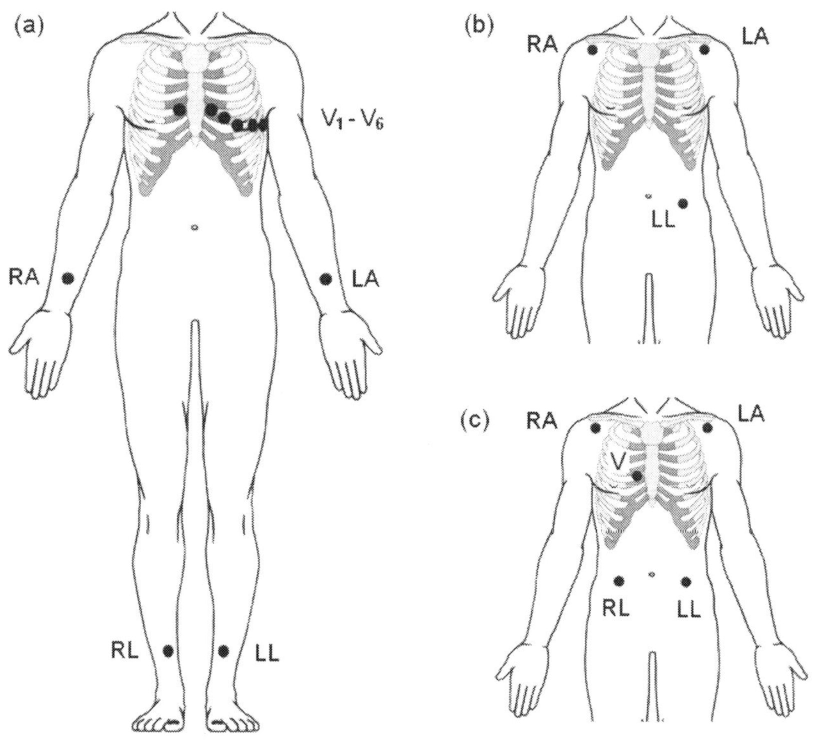

Figure 2-1 Electrode placements for three types of ECG monitoring. (a) 12-lead ECG. (b) 3-lead ECG. (c) 5-lead ECG. (Modified from [25]).

3-lead ECGs tend to be monitored continuously and viewed on the screen of an appropriate monitoring device, for example during an operation or whilst being transported in an ambulance [26, 27]. Usually, a wireless ECG monitoring system is used to continuously monitor one or two most informative ECG signals, and in most cases, 3-lead ECG measurement configured is used.

As shown in Figure 2-2 (a), a 3-lead ECG system can be used to acquire three recognized potential difference signals across the thorax, and they are usually called Lead I, Lead II and Lead III, respectively. Lead I is the potential difference between the anatomical right arm and the anatomical left arm, while Lead II and Lead III are potential differences between anatomical right arm and anatomical left leg, and between anatomical left arm and anatomical left leg, respectively. Figure 2-2 (b) shows a typical Lead II ECG waveform that clearly depicts the classical components of an ECG waveform, including P wave, QRS complex, and T and U waves. Diagnostically relevant quantities, including PR interval, QRS duration, ST segment duration, T wave amplitude (referred as T wave alternant) and T wave width can be obtained directly from the ECG waveform. The derived quantities of interest mainly include R peak to R peak interval (RRI), variability in ST segment duration and amplitude, and power spectrum and wavelet domain analysis of heart rate variability (HRV) sequences obtained from (RRI).

RRI is the time elapsed between the onset of an R peak of the ECG and that of the next, so it signifies the time between two consecutive beats, and is often used for heart rate determination and arrythmic cardiac activity detection. The variability of RRI is referred to as heart rate variability (HRV). A human RRI series has three major frequency components: (i) the very low frequency (VLF), (ii) the low frequency (LF) around 0.1 Hz, and (iii) the high frequency (HF) between 0.2 Hz and

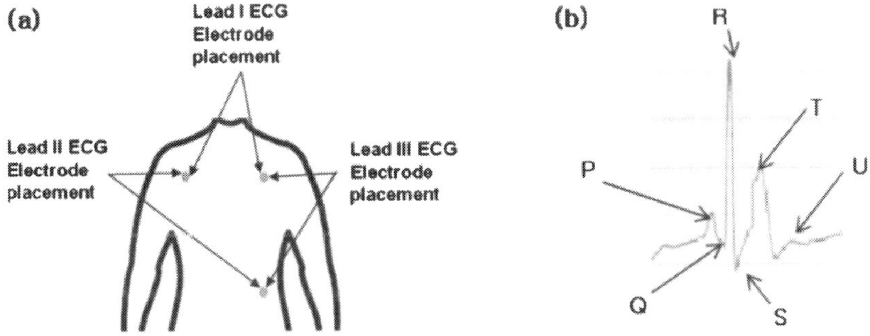

Figure 2-2 A 3-lead ECG Measurement. (a) Electrode placement for a 3-lead ECG measurement. (b) A typical Lead II ECG waveform with the characteristic P wave, QRS complex, and T and U waves.

0.4 Hz. The algorithms for extracting RRI involve an identification of the instances of the R-wave occurrence or of the QRS complex in the ECG data, followed by concatenating the time-differences between successive instances. The RRI series is rich in information about the cardiovascular physiology of a subject.

Although there is some disagreement with respect to the physiological indication of the LF component, most studies consider LF to be an indicator of sympathetic nerve modulation of heart rate. The HF reflects vagal nerve influence on the same. The ratio LF/HF is used as a diagnostic quantity that can reflect the autonomic neuropathy due to chronic diseases such as diabetes. A reduction in this ratio has been observed in the case of postmyocardial infarction patients. A lower HRV has been shown to be indicative of compromised cardiac health. Thus HRV analysis has been studied as a valuable, noninvasive and easy to implement diagnostic tool. However, it is important to note that factors such as fiducial point selection for HRV calculation, sampling rate, and considerations of data latency are the key to obtaining reproducible results.

Complete cardiac monitoring requires real time ECG for the detection of arrhythmic heart beats, ST segment abnormalities associated with ischemic attacks, myocardial infarction, and other waveform characteristics such as PR interval and QRS complex width. These are indicative of the functioning of the atria of the heart and blockages in the cardiac electric conduction pathways, respectively. HRV analysis, on the other hand, provides insight into changes in the regulation of cardiovascular function stemming from chronic diseases such as diabetes and hypertension, which are major risk factors for the occurrence of cardiovascular diseases (CVDs). Techniques like HRV analysis through time, frequency, and wavelet domain analysis techniques have been successful in tracking autonomic nervous-cardiovascular regulation, which is indicative of chronic diseases. Thus, various parameters derivable from ECG are of significant prognostic value with regard to CVDs.

2.1.2 Electroencephalogram (EEG)

(1) Basic characteristics of EEG

A brain whispers messages to the body through electrical impulses transmitted to the central nervous system. If the brain is injured, these electrical impulses or brain waves may be disturbed, resulting in abnormal rhythmic patterns. When the brain continues to transmit these abnormal patterns, imbalances are created in the body. Neural signal communication is achieved by the production and propagation of small electrical signals produced by the nerve cells called neurons. Electroencephalography is a medical imaging technique that reads scalp electrical activity generated by brain structures. EEG is an electrical activity, which is recorded from the scalp surface with the help of metal electrodes and conductive gel.

When neurons (brain cells) are activated, local current flows are produced. Differences in electrical potentials are caused by summing postsynaptic graded potentials from pyramidical cells that create electrical dipoles between soma (body of neuron) and apical dendrites. The electrical activity of the brain is recorded with different kinds of electrode placements (scalp, cortical, and depth).

As discussed above, the origin of EEG is due to the firing of the neurons and the post-synaptic potential that is generated after the neuron firing. The transfer of information from one neuron to another neuron occurs across a synapse, which is a small gap separating neurons. The synapse consists of a presynaptic ending containing neuron-transmitters, a post-synaptic ending that contains receptor sites for neurotransmitters and a synaptic cleft or space between the presynaptic and post-synaptic endings. The amplitude of this evoked potential is generally very small. The signal measured on the scalp is further reduced in amplitude due to various factors such as the skull, the layer of fat present for protecting the brain, hair on the scalp as well as the skin. Hence, the amplitude of EEG is generally in the range of 0.1–100 mV [28].

To perform an EEG recording, electrodes with wires designed to detect electrical signals are attached on the scalp with special adhesives. The electrodes are placed in pairs so that the difference in electric potential between them can be measured. Although the basic EEG pattern remains a standard, it varies from person to person and every individual has his own unique EEG pattern. The EEG changes with brain disorder, such as epilepsy, so it can be a useful diagnostic tool but usually must be accompanied by other diagnostic tests [29]. The most common electrical activities of the brain are summarized in Figure 2-3 and Table 2-1.

(2) Principle for EEG measurement

When a neuron firing takes place, an action potential is generated at the presynaptic end and at the post-synaptic end, and an evoked potential is generated, which is the source of an electroencephalogram. Thousands of neurons fire in a human brain and an EEG signal can be detected on the scalp. These signals are obtained at a very low frequency of the order of less than 60 Hz. Synapses are crucial to the biological computations that underlie perception and thought. They also provide the means through which the nervous system connects to and controls the other systems of the body. A human brain contains a huge number of such chemical synapses.

The EEG signal is a parameter of consciousness of a person. As the neuron activity in the brain increases, the EEG shifts to a higher dominating frequency and a lower amplitude. When the eyes are closed, the alpha waves begin to dominate the EEG. When a person falls asleep, the dominant EEG frequency decreases. In some cases, rapid eye movements can be observed when a person dreams. In deep sleep, the EEG has large and slow deflections

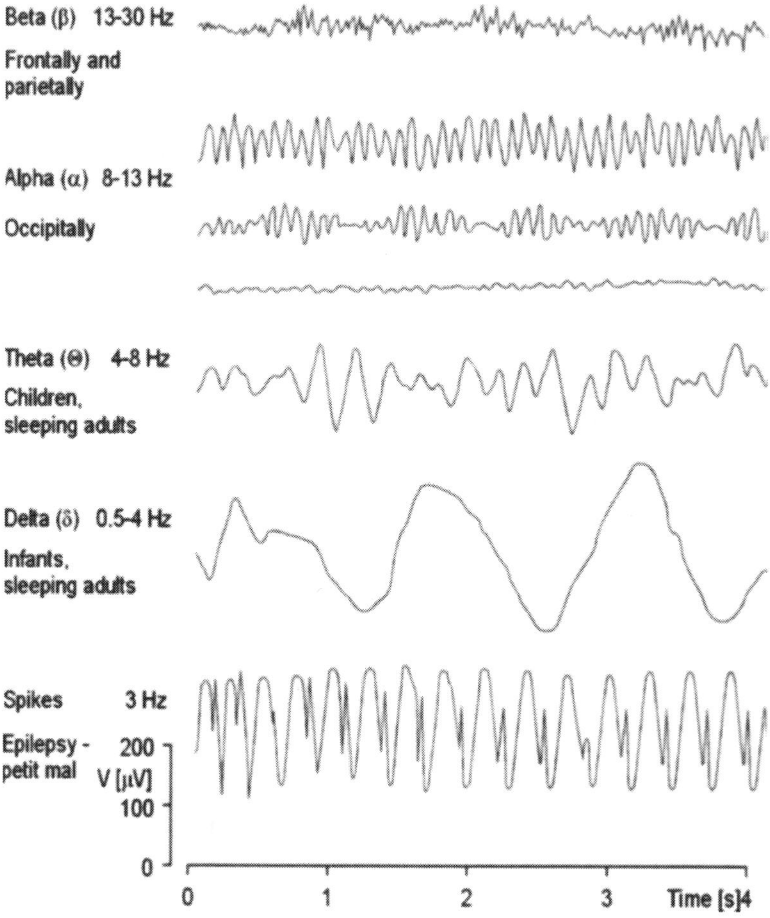

Figure 2-3 Waveforms representing various EEG signals at different frequencies [29].

called delta waves. No cerebral activity can be detected from a patient with complete cerebral death.

In clinical electroencephalography, twenty one (21) electrodes are applied to the head in what is known as the 10–20 system as shown in Figure 2-4. To record the electrical activity in the brain, the location of the electrodes on the scalp is very important. Scalp electrodes are placed in conjunction with both monopolar as well as bipolar configurations. With the monopolar configuration, one side of each amplifier is connected to a reference electrode, often located on the ear lobe. With the bipolar recording configuration, the amplifiers are connected between pairs of scalp electrodes in a regular order. More data can be obtained with bipolar scalp-to-scalp recordings.

Table 2-1. Possible source of activity in certain EEG frequency band. (Source: Lonkar, M., 2006, *Design, Fabrication and Implementation of Compact Amplifiers for Ambulatory EEG (electroencephalogram) Monitoring*, M. Sc. thesis, University of Arkansas.)

Electrical activity	Frequency of occurrence	Characteristics
Beta activity	13–30 Hz frontal and parietal lobe	Normal activity, present when the eyes are open or closed. Some drugs increase the amount of beta activity in the EEG.
Alpha activity	8–13 Hz occipital lobe	Also, a normal activity, present in waking adults. It is only seen when the eyes are closed and should disappear or reduce in amplitude when the eyes are open.
Theta activity	4–8 Hz back and central areas of the brain	It can be classed as both a normal and abnormal activity depending on the age and state of the patient. In adults, it is normal if the patient is drowsy. However, it can also indicate brain dysfunction if it is seen in a patient who is alert and awake.
Delta activity	0.5–4 Hz	It is only normal in an adult patient if he is in a moderate to deep sleep. If it is seen at any other time, it would indicate brain dysfunction. Abnormal activity may be seen in all or some channels depending on the underlying brain problem.
Spike and wave activity	Random frequency <60 Hz	Number of other waveforms, which are more specific to certain conditions. For example, spike and wave activity indicates a seizure disorder. Other epileptic conditions may be diagnosed if spikes or sharp waves are seen.

The 10–20 system is based on the relationship between the location of an electrode and the underlying area of cerebral cortex. Every point in Figure 2-4 indicates a possible electrode position. Each site has a letter (to identify the lobe) and a number or another letter to identify the hemisphere location. The letters F, T, C, P, and O stand for frontal, temporal, central, parietal, and occipital, respectively. The even numbers (2, 4, 6, and 8) refer to the right hemisphere

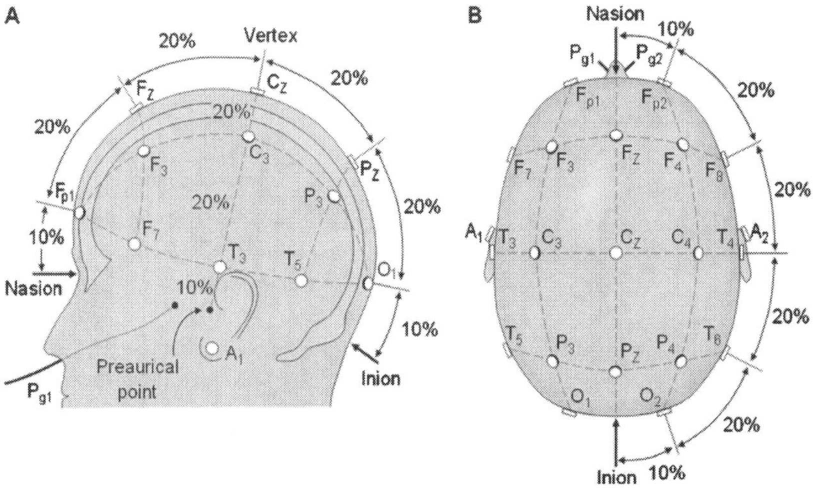

Figure 2-4 Labels for points according to 10–20 systems of electrodes placement [29].

and the odd numbers (1, 3, 5, and 7) refer to the left hemisphere. The letter "z" refers to an electrode placed on the midline of the scalp. The smaller the number, the closer the position is to the midline. The EEG recording is taken by attaching 16–25 silver or gold cup electrodes along with a conductive media to different places on the head. These electrodes are connected to the amplifier by wires that amplify and record the electrical activity inside the brain. The amplitude signal is given to a data acquisition unit and the electrical activity is recorded for analysis. Table 2-2 shows the clinical setup for an EEG.

Table 2-2. Clinical setup for an EEG. (Source: Lonkar, M., 2006, *Design, Fabrication and Implementation of Compact Amplifiers for Ambulatory EEG (electroencephalogram) Monitoring*, M. Sc. thesis, University of Arkansas.)

Resources required	Electrodes, electrode gel, EEG module and amplifier, power supply, portable computer, waveform analysis software.
Material consumed	Electrolytes and silver/gold electrodes.
Electrode placement	A pair of electrodes (Ag–AgCl) are placed in the scalp, following the 10–20 electrode placement system.
Measurement procedure	The signal obtained from the electrodes placed on the scalp, which is amplified by an appropriate biopotential amplifier and recorded preferably on computer.
Range of values	Depends on individual subjects, time source, and recording position used.

2.1.3 Arterial pulse wave and pulse transit time

At the end of each cardiac cycle, fresh oxygenated blood from the left ventricle is pumped into the aorta through the semilunar valves in the heart. The periodic contraction of the left ventricle to pump blood into the aorta results in the pulsatile flow of blood in the arteries. This pulsatile flow is described as the arterial pulse wave. The average velocity of propagation of this pulse wave from the heart to the peripheral arteries of the body is called the arterial pressure pulse wave. The arterial pulse wave gives information about both the traveling wave towards the peripheral arteries as well as the reflected wave from the periphery. The changes that occur in the flow wave can form an important metric for assessing age-related stiffening of the arteries in cases like systolic hypertension [30]. Studies have been performed on the diagnostic value of harmonic analysis of arterial pressure pulse wave as well [31].

The pulse transit time (PPT) is defined as the time elapsed between the ejection of blood from the heart and the arrival of the arterial pressure pulse at a peripheral artery. The most popular fiducial points for determining PPT have been the R peak of the ECG waveform and the upward slope of the pulse waveform. The main reason for this choice is that the R peaks can be easily detected. This method assumes that the time period between the occurrence of the R peak and the actual ejection of blood from the heart, referred as pre-ejection period (PEP), is constant. As will be further discussed in Section 2.4, good estimates of blood pressure can be made despite the discounting of PEP [32].

2.2 Bioelectric sensors based on carbon nanotubes

To record biolectric signals of a patient using a current health monitoring systems, electrodes are attached to the skin of the patient, and conductive gel is used to ensure the electrical connection between the electrodes and the skin. The electrode wires are connected to a processing recording system. The subject has to be in close proximity of these machines due to the direct electrical connections with the body and the machine. The conductive gel along with many wires connected to the bioelectric electrodes makes them uncomfortable for the subject, making the recording and monitoring of the patient's sleep patterns very difficult. The patient has to be in a sleep lab and/or a hospital at all times and at least one technician needs to watch the patient's sleep behavior via video. The patient can not experience normal sleep patterns under such environments, and so the diagnostic results are not really very conclusive. The commonly monitored bioelectric signals are ECG, EEG, EMG, and EOG. The electrodes for monitoring these signals are Ag/AgCl and gold, which require skin preparation by means of scrubbing to remove the dead cells and application of electrolytic gel to reduce the skin contact resistance. The electrolytic gel reduces the contact impedance between the skin and the conventional Ag/AgCl electrode. However, the wet conventional Ag/AgCl electrode has drawbacks such as skin irritations and the difficulty in long time monitoring because the gel dries out after a few hours. Usually, physiological parameters are monitored over an extended period of time during the patient's normal daily life to diagnose a disease. In this case, the wet conventional Ag/AgCl cannot be used because of the dry-out of gel. The dry-out of gel increases the impedance between the skin and the electrode, greatly decreasing the signal sensitivity. Also noises, such as motion artifact and baseline wander, are added to the bioelectric signals as the electrode floats over the electrolytic gel during the monitoring period. To overcome these drawbacks, dry nanoelectrodes are preferable because good electrical contact can be established by holding dry nanoelectrodes to the skin surface without the need for electrolytic fluids or gels. Because the sensitivity of an electrode is related to its surface area, a dry nanoelectrode can be much more sensitive than a conventional dry electrode due to its large surface area.

Carbon nanotube (CNT)-based dry electrodes are promising candidates for bioelectric signal recording [33]. Usually a CNT-based electrode is made by mixing multiwall carbon nanotubes with epoxy and then pasting the composite on the surface of electrode substrate. In order to enhance electrode performance, the surface of the CNT composite should be activated. Figure 2-5 shows the comparison between a CNT composite electrode and a plasma-treated CNT composite electrode.

Several electrodes for bioelectric recording are shown in Figure 2-6, including Ag/AgCl, carbon nanotube composite, plasma-treated carbon nanotube composite, and gold nanowire electrodes. To compare their sensitivities, these electrodes are attached on the forehead to sense the bioelectric signals with eye movement (blinking), and the electrode-skin-electrode-impedance (ESEI) and EOG were measured. Figure 2-7 shows the experiment setup. The wireless system was used to monitor and save the data in real time.

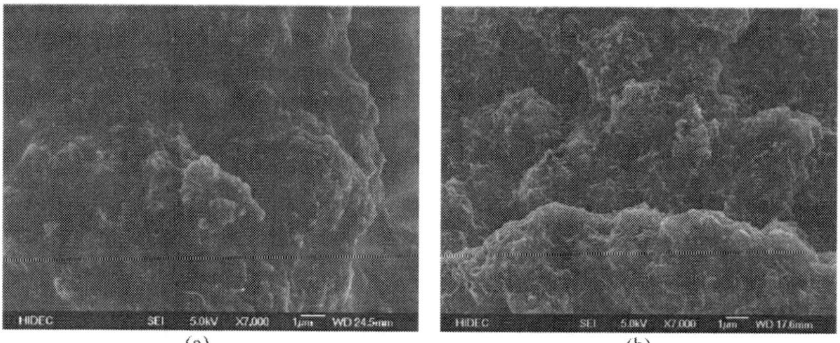

(a) (b)

Figure 2-5 Comparison between a CNT composite electrode and a plasma-treated CNT composite electrode. (a) SEM image of a CNT composite electrode. (b) SEM image of plasma-treated CNT composite electrode.

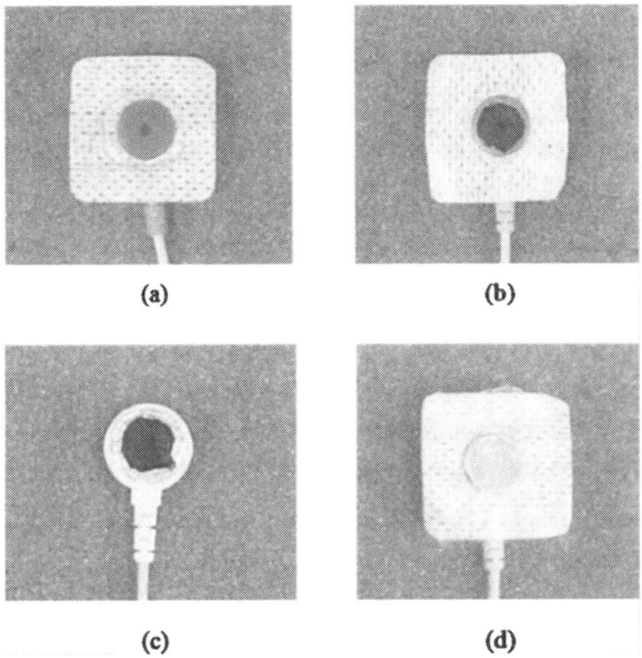

Figure 2-6 Electrodes for bioelectric recording. (a) Conventional wet Ag/AgCl electrode, (b) carbon nanotube electrode, (c) plasma treated carbon nanotube electrode, and (d) gold nanowire electrode.

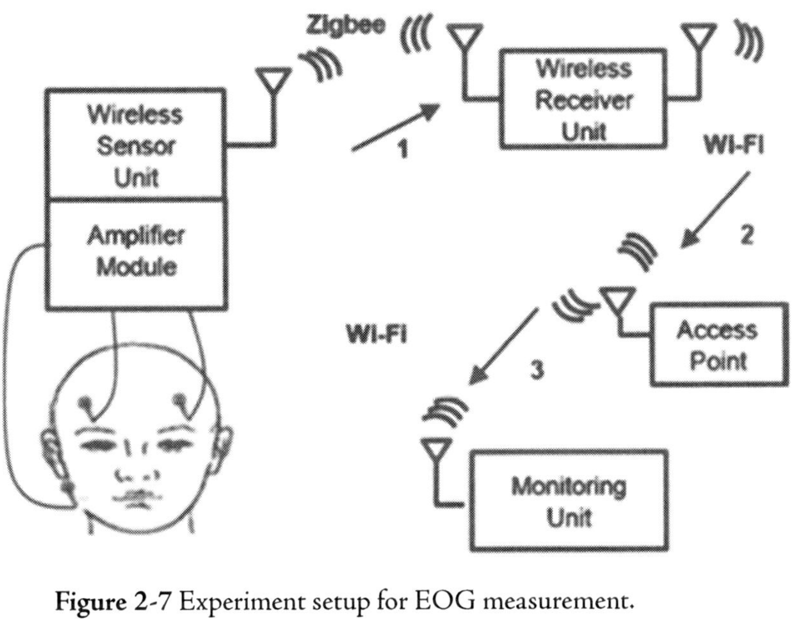

Figure 2-7 Experiment setup for EOG measurement.

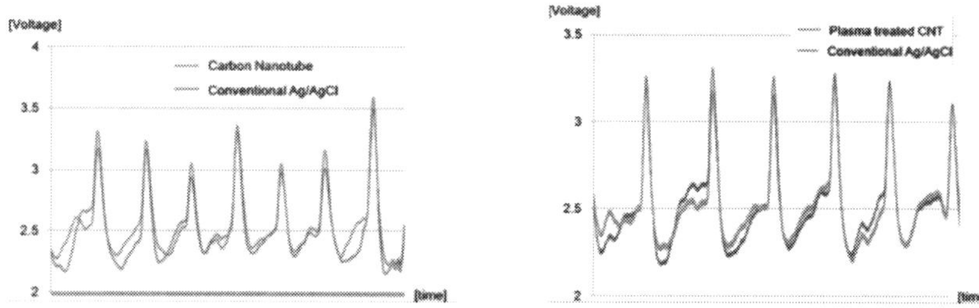

(a) (b)

Figure 2-8 Measurement results of EOG with different electrodes. (a) EOG signals with carbon nanotube and wet Ag/AgCl electrodes. (b) EOG signals with plasma treated carbon nanotube and wet Ag/AgCl electrodes

The signals from the sensor unit were transmitted to the monitoring unit through the receiver unit.

Figure 2-8 shows the bioelectric signals obtained by using conventional wet Ag/AgCl electrodes, CNT electrodes and plasma treated CNT electrodes [33]. It is found that the sensitivity of the plasma treated CNT electrodes is higher than that of the conventional wet Ag/AgCl electrode by 7.7%. Here the sensitivity is defined as the peak-to-peak amplitude of the signals from a conventional Ag/AgCl, carbon nanotube, and plasma-treated carbon nanotube electrodes under the same test conditions.

2.3 Bioelectric sensors based on metal nanowires

To overcome the drawbacks of conventional electrodes with gel, Au nanowire electrodes were developed [33]. Vertically aligned Au nanowire arrays were fabricated for EEG dry electrodes. These electrodes have a brush-like structure, consisting of vertically aligned conducting nanostructure supported over a conducting substrate. Figure 2-9 shows the SEM image of vertically aligned Au nanowires.

To measure the biopotential signals of eye movement, three gold nanowire electrodes are placed on the forehead along the horizontal axis. Also a reference electrode is placed on the backside of earlobe, acting as the body ground. The movement of eye ball is classified as five motions: blinking, left, right, up, and down movements. Figure 2-10 indicates that there is a change in the phase of the angle depending upon the direction of rotation of the eye. It justifies that the signal generated is proportional to the sine of the angle of rotation of the eye ball. It can be noticed that there is a variation in the amplitude of the channels depending on the location of the electrodes. Also, there may be a slight variation in the noise level depending upon the body impedance. However, the major variation in each channel is due to the difference in eye movement, such as different rotation of the eye ball.

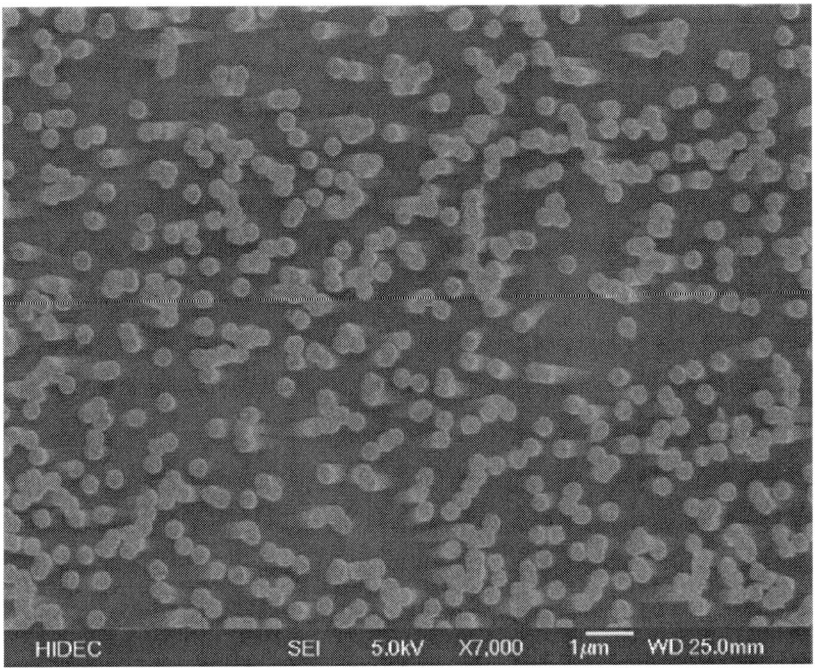

Figure 2-9 SEM image of 2 μm long vertically aligned Au nanowires grown by template method.

To confirm the advantages of gold nanowire electrodes in biopotential measurement, these are placed on proper locations to sense EOG, EMG, and EEG, as shown in Figure 2-11 [33]. A five-channel wireless POC system was used to monitor and save data in real time. Figure 2-12 (a) shows the EOG measurement results. The gold nanowire electrodes, which are placed on the right lower and left upper side of the eyes, detected EOG with the eye motion, blinks, up, down, left, and right movement. EMG is detected by a gold nanowire electrode with the movement of chin as shown in Figure 2-12 (b). EEG was measured at the C3 and O2 position. The C3 position is a part of parietal lobe and the O2 position is a part of occipital lobe of brain. Figure 2-12 (c) shows that beta waves are presented in the C3 position and alpha waves appeared when the eyes were closed and reduced in amplitude when the eyes are open in the O2 position. In addition, ECG was also measured. As shown in Figure 2-12 (d), P wave, QRS complex, and T wave, the components of ECG, were sensed with the dry gold nanowires electrodes.

Figure 2-12 indicates that, due to its large surface area and high conductivity, the vertically aligned Au nanowire electrode is sensitive enough to measure biopotential signals, which are usually in the range of 0.1–100 mV [33].

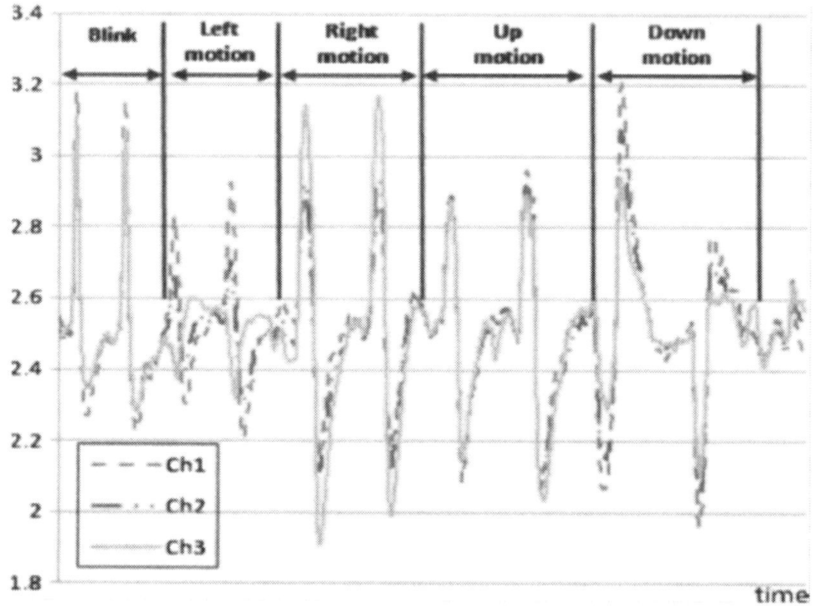

Figure 2-10 The biopotential signals measured with gold nanowire electrodes. The three channels correspond to the three electrodes placed on the forehead.

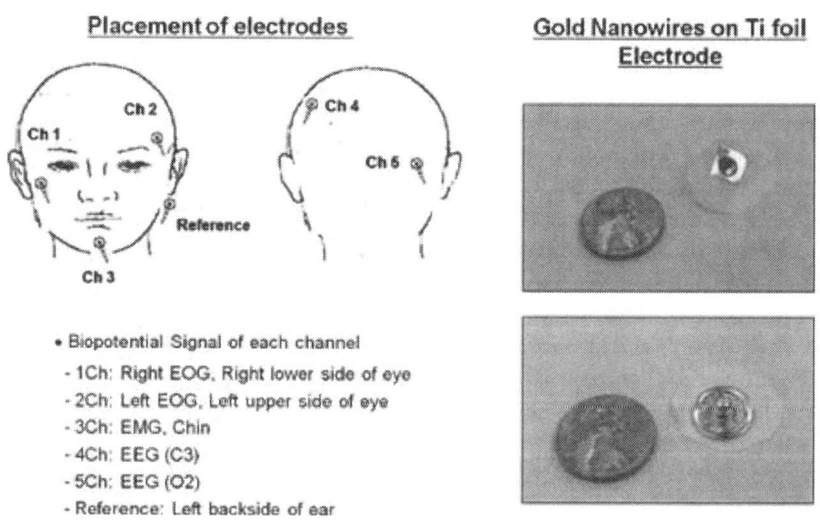

Figure 2-11 Biopotentials test set up for dry gold nanowire electrodes.

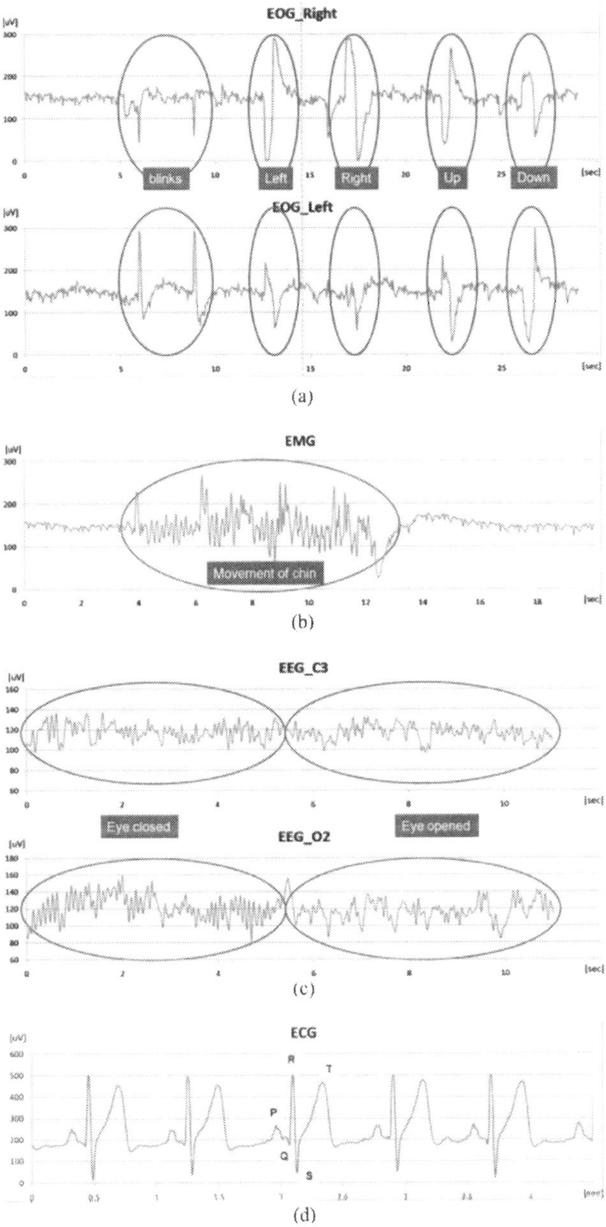

Figure 2-12 Measurement results of bio-potential signals.
(a) EOG measurements with dry gold nanowire electrodes.
(b) EMG measurements with dry gold nanowire electrodes.
(c) EEG measurements with dry gold nanowire electrodes.
(d) ECG measurements with dry gold nanowire electrodes.

2.4 Cuffless blood pressure sensors

In this method, the blood pressure is derived from the time elapsed between the contraction of the left ventricle and the detection of pulse at a peripheral artery [34]. The time of the contraction of the left ventricle is determined by ECG measurement, and the pulse at the peripheral artery is detected by an arterial pulse wave sensor.

The primary relation between pulse wave velocity (PWV) and coefficient of elasticity (E) of the artery vessel walls is given by the Moens-Korteweg equation [35]. The pulse transit time (PTT) is measured by the time elapsed between the origin of the pulse wave at the heart, corresponding to the contraction of the ventricle, and the detection of the pulse wave in a peripheral artery. PTT has been used as a metric for arterial wall stiffness resulting from stenosis and arteriosclerosis and as an indirect means of measuring the blood pressure. Following the mathematical development described in [32], we have:

$$\mathrm{PWV} = \frac{L}{T} = \sqrt{\frac{tE_0 e^{\alpha P}}{\rho d}} \tag{1}$$

where PWV is the arterial pulse wave velocity, L is the length of the arterial path from the left ventricle to the radial artery at the wrist, T is the time elapsed between the contraction of the left ventricle and the detection of pulse at a peripheral artery, t is the thickness of the vessel, ρ is the density of blood, d is the diameter of the vessel, $E_0 e^{\alpha P}$ is the pressure dependent Young's modulus of the artery, α is a constant dependent on the vessel and P is the blood pressure [5]. By taking the Young's modulus, diameter, length and thickness of the artery as constants with minimal variability, Eq. (1) becomes [34, 36]:

$$P = \frac{2}{\alpha}\left(\ln L - \ln T - \frac{1}{2}\ln k\right) = \left(\frac{-2}{\alpha}\right)\ln T + Const. \tag{2}$$

with k given by:

$$k = \sqrt{\frac{tE_0}{\rho d}} \tag{3}$$

Eq. (2) indicates that as PTT increases the blood pressure decreases and vice versa.

The sensor for arterial pressure pulse was a 110 micron thick, uniaxially oriented, metallized PVDF film. The PVDF film exhibits charge separation due to the piezoelectric nature of PVDF when subjected to radial strain perpendicular to the direction of polling. The dome shaped silicone rubber enclosure, as illustrated in Figure 2-13, converts the vertical force applied by the arterial pressure pulse at the wrist into a radial deformation in the film. Electrical contacts to both surfaces of the PVDF films are made using conductive silver epoxy and enamel coated stainless steel wires which were

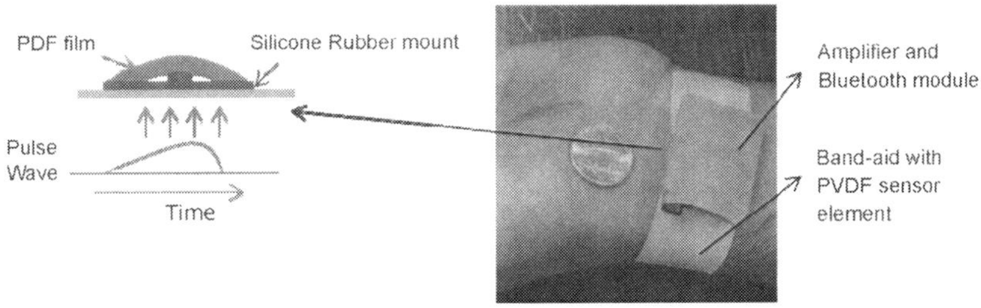

Figure 2-13 Mounting of PVDF film sensor to detect the arterial pressure pulse wave.

integrated in the Band-aid. Connections between the wireless module and the sensor are made through standard snap-on buttons.

For PTT measurement, the time elapsed was determined between the R peak of the ECG which corresponds to the depolarization of the left ventricle and the peak of the pulse wave detected at the wrist, as shown in Figure 2-14. The ECG sensors using gold nanowires were mounted in the Lead I position. Data from both sensors were acquired simultaneously at a Bluetooth enabled PC and the pulse transit times were calculated. Blood pressure readings from a validated OMRON HEM 712C (OMRON Corporation, Shimogyo-ku, Kyoto, Japan) were used to build the calibration relationship between the experimentally calculated PTTs and systolic blood pressure [34].

The flow chart for the program implemented on the PC for PTT extraction is also shown in Figure 2-14. There are two sensors in the experimental setup: one for pulse wave and one for ECG. The data read from both sensors were parsed on the PC and fed to a peak detection algorithm: R peak in case

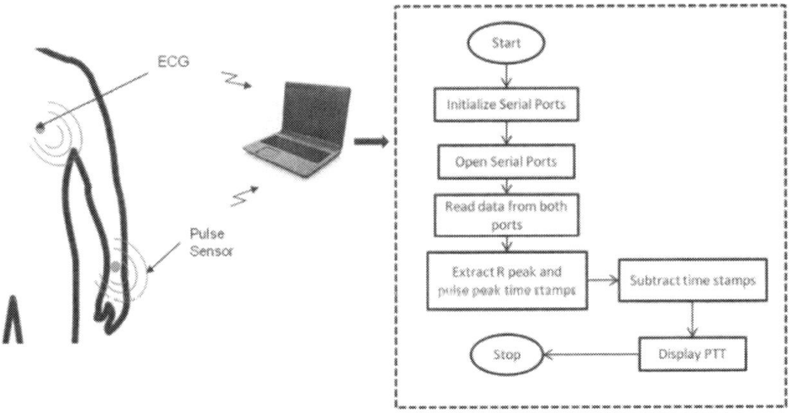

Figure 2-14 The experimental setup and the algorithm for PTT extraction.

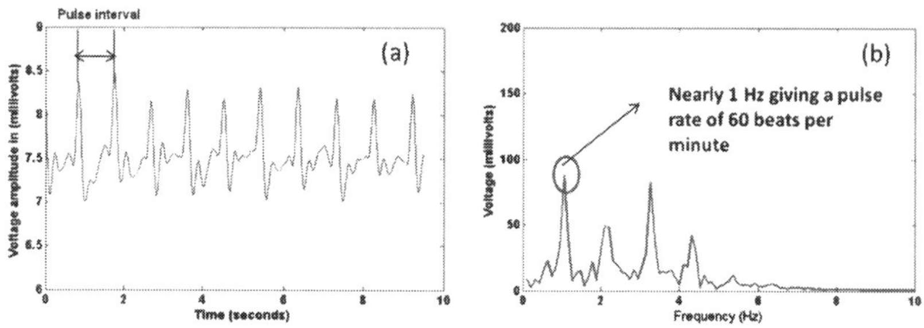

Figure 2-15 (a) Pulse waveform obtained at the wrist over 10 seconds (b) The Fast Fourier transform of the pulse waveform in (a).

of ECG and pulse peak in case of pressure pulse wave. The peak detection algorithm gives the sequence of time stamps at which peaks were detected and simple array subtraction of the R peak time stamps from the pulse time stamps gives the PTT in units of inverse of sampling rate.

The inverse of the time elapsed between the peaks of the pulse waveforms gives the pulse rate. The use of amplitude based threshold techniques to detect the peaks is the most straightforward but tracking of the first fundamental peak in the frequency spectrum is immune to signals corrupted with 60 Hz powerline noise. Figure 2-15 shows the data obtained from the pulse rate sensor module at the level of the wrist.

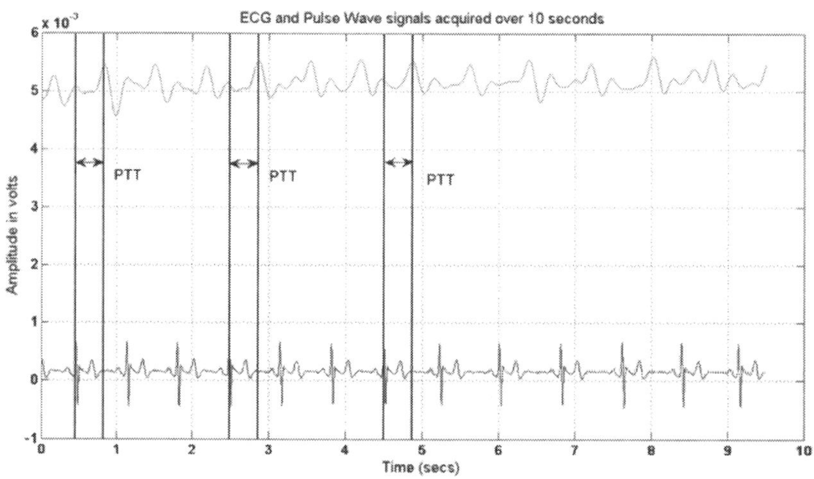

Figure 2-16 Pulse transit time as observed in a simultaneous plot of ECG and pulse pressure wave from the wrist.

In the experiments, the fiducial point for ECG was the R peak and the fiducial point for the pulse pressure wave was the peak of the waveform, for each heartbeat. The PTT calculation is illustrated in Figure 2-16.

The PTT obtained from 10 second long sets of data were matched with corresponding readings taken from the OMRON pressure cuff measurement. Ten readings were taken as an initial measure of accuracy from a 23 year old, healthy individual with no prior cardiac abnormalities. The natural logarithms of the PTTs were plotted against the measured systolic blood pressure. A linear fit was then calculated between the logarithm of PTT and systolic blood pressure to reveal a linear relation with a negative slope. Figure 2-17 shows the curve fit for the data.

The low R-square fit obtained may be explained by the small data set that was used. However, the expected trend of increased blood pressure with reduced PTT is observable and establishes the feasibility of using multiple independent sensors for simultaneous acquisition. However, the PVDF used in the system is not biodegradable and its cost is high. Electroactive paper made with cellulose is an environmentally friendly and cheap alternative that can be used to replace PVDF in this application [37].

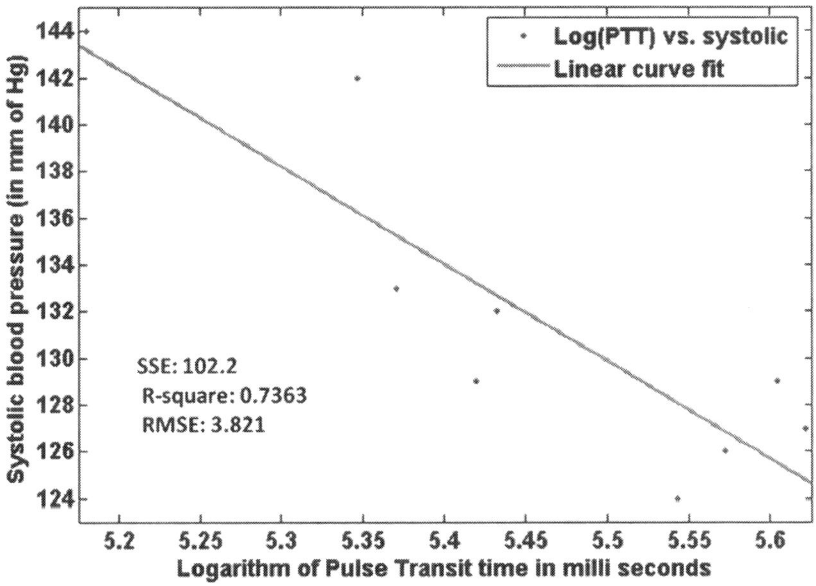

Figure 2-17 The linear fit between measured systolic blood pressure and estimated PTT.

3. Telecommunication and information technologies for mobile health monitoring systems

3.1 Introduction

Telecommunication and information technologies play important roles in the development of mobile health monitoring systems. The wireless communication system of a mobile health monitoring system mainly consists of three units: a wireless sensor unit, a wireless receiver, and a monitoring unit. The wireless sensor unit is used for detecting signals and transmitting signals to the wireless receiver module. The wireless receiver unit is used as a repeater. It receives the signals from the sensor unit module and transmits the signals to the monitoring unit or remote server.

In the following, the design of wireless transmitter and wireless receiver are discussed with examples. Smartphones are discussed subsequently as a special type of receivers. Following this, an example of the wireless communication system, e-Nanoflex, is discussed.

3.2 Wireless transmitter unit

A wireless transmitter unit mainly consists of sensors, an amplifier module, a process board, a power management board, and a wireless module [38]. The main functions of the process board include changing analog signals to digital signals (AD conversion) and managing the data flow from acquisition to transmission. As the outputs of the sensor have small amplitudes ranging from a few μV to a few mV, containing undesirable signals, such as noises from power line interface (50 Hz/60 Hz) and thermal noise, amplification and filtration are needed before they are sent to the AD convertor (ADC). Another role of the amplifier module is to adjust the signal level to the input range of the ADC (0–5 V).

In data acquisition, accurate sampling of the input analog signals at the desired frequency and creating data packets with provisions for reliable transmission should be considered. In the wireless data transmission, in addition to considering the basic specification of wireless communication standards, such as power consumption, throughput and coverage, the interface type between a wireless module and a processor should be considered to guarantee the throughput because not only the data rate of a wireless module but also the data transfer rate of the interface restrict the throughput of the whole system. Because the wireless transmitter unit is a portable device and acts like a sensor node or a slave, its key factors are low power consumption, low cost, and the number of sensor nodes connected to a gateway or a master.

Figure 3-1 shows the block diagram and the picture of a wireless transmitter unit. A Zigbee wireless module is used to communicate between the transmitter and the receiver unit, and the frequency band of the Zigbee module is the 2.4 GHz industrial, scientific, and medical (ISM) band. Zigbee is in the spotlight

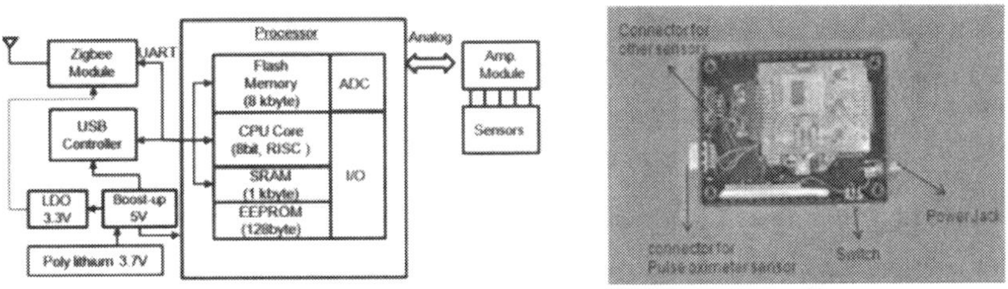

(a) (b)

Figure 3-1 Wireless transmitter unit. (a) Block diagram, (b) picture.

in a wireless sensor network. First, Zigbee can support many sensor nodes by building network topology with a start, a cluster tree, or a mesh network, which makes it easy to extend a network widely. The second feature of Zigbee is its low power consumption. Because the wake-up time of Zigbee is the shortest among the current wireless standards, it can keep power consumption low by changing alternately the status between the sleep and wake-up modes. In addition, considering cost and data rate, Zigbee is the best choice for a wireless sensor network. Since the Zigbee module provides an integrated command and serial communications to handle a processor, the need for external modulation/demodulation and external protocol handling by the host controller is not needed. The power for the wireless transmitter unit shown in Figure 3.1 (b) is provided by a 3.7 V poly-lithium battery. A voltage regulator steps up the voltage to 5 V. The regulated 5.0 V is supplied to the microprocessor and the amplifier module. The 5.0 V voltage steps down to the 3.3 V by another voltage regulator, and the 3.3 V is used for operating the Zigbee module [38].

3.3 Wireless receiver unit

A wireless receiver unit receives data from the transmitter unit and transmits the data to the monitoring system [38]. As Zigbee is not yet prevalent, it is not suitable to be used in building a remote network. Using a widespread wireless standard, Wi-Fi, is more cost effective in building a remote network. The wireless receiver unit enables the signals to be monitored in remote places by Wi-Fi and the Ethernet network. Therefore, the wireless transmitter unit builds a local sensor network with Zigbee, and the wireless receiver unit builds an extended sensor network, a remote monitoring network with Wi-Fi.

Figure 3.2 shows the block diagram and image of the wireless receiver unit. The wireless receiver unit consists of a Zigbee module, a Wi-Fi module, and a processor board, which has two external 16 Mbyte synchronous dynamic random access memory (SDRAM), a 64 Mbyte Nand Flash memory, and a microprocessor. The memories are needed to process and store data. SDRAM is used as the buffer for the sensor data, and the flash memory

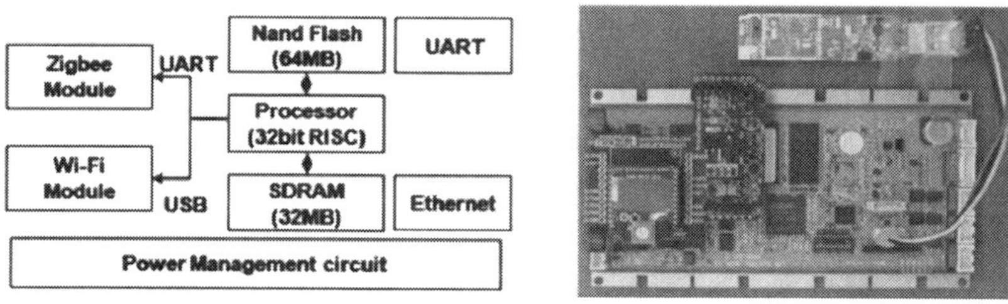

Figure 3-2 Wireless receiver unit. (a) Block diagram, (b) image.

is used for the storage of programs. In addition, the receiver unit has the Ethernet controller so that it can be connected to the Ethernet network.

The wireless receiver unit has two wireless modules: one is a Zigbee module to receive data from the wireless sensor unit and the other is a Wi-Fi module to transmit data to the central monitoring system through the Internet. The Zigbee RF module used was the same model used in the wireless sensor unit to eliminate the possible interoperation problems. Because the receiver unit adopts the most widespread wireless standard, Wi-Fi, the sensed signal can be transmitted through a large number of hot spots. Wi-Fi also has the advantages of wide range coverage (100 m) and the high data rate (54 Mbit/s). The Wi-Fi module is connected to the microprocessor through the universal serial bus (USB) interface. Since it can support a high data transmission rate, data can be transferred to the monitoring unit in a short time, compared with other wireless standards. Furthermore, it provides an easy way to construct the sensor network through the prevalent Internet network [33]. A 5.0 V adaptor is used to supply power to the unit instead of a battery because the receiver unit is used as a stationary device. Three types of voltage regulators are used to provide appropriate voltages to each component. The 3.3 V is for the Zigbee module, external memories, and I/O ports of microprocessor. The 2.7 V and 1.2 V are for the internal memories and the microprocessor, respectively [38].

3.4 Smartphone

Smartphones have a number of key features that make them advantageous over other information and communication technologies in particular activities in healthcare [20, 39]. Firstly, Smartphones have wireless cellular communication capability, providing the potential for continuous, interactive communication from any locations, for example telephone calls, text and multimedia messaging and also internet access. Secondly, they are portable because of their small size, low weight, and rechargeable and long-life battery power. Thirdly, they have sufficient computing power to support software applications. Further, global positioning system (GPS) and location-enabled Smartphones offer many additional application opportunities that can further assist the independent living of persons with disabilities and multiple chronic conditions.

The potential for Smartphones to transform healthcare is tremendous. The use of a Smartphone as a base station for receiving data offers the advantage of cellular network connectivity to the Internet [40]. Further, the strong computing capability of modern Smartphones has made it possible to develop a system where automated analysis is done in the phone, and only the parts of the data where the analysis application would find abnormalities will be sent to the server for further analysis [41]. Due to the rapid developments in embedded computing and the emergence of Smartphones as powerful portable computing devices, truly pervasive computing could be realized.

The application of Smartphones in mobile health monitoring systems is further discussed in Section 3.5.3, where technical details are given.

3.5 e-Nanoflex

In this section, the e-Nanoflex system [18] is discussed as an example of wireless communication and data processing system. Besides its hardware architecture, the issues related to data transfer, storage and processing will be discussed.

3.5.1 Hardware architecture

The e-Nanoflex system comprises of a sensor and the supporting hardware peripherals for data acquisition. As schematically shown in Figure 3-3, the sensor, amplifier and filter circuits for conditioning the sensor signal, the

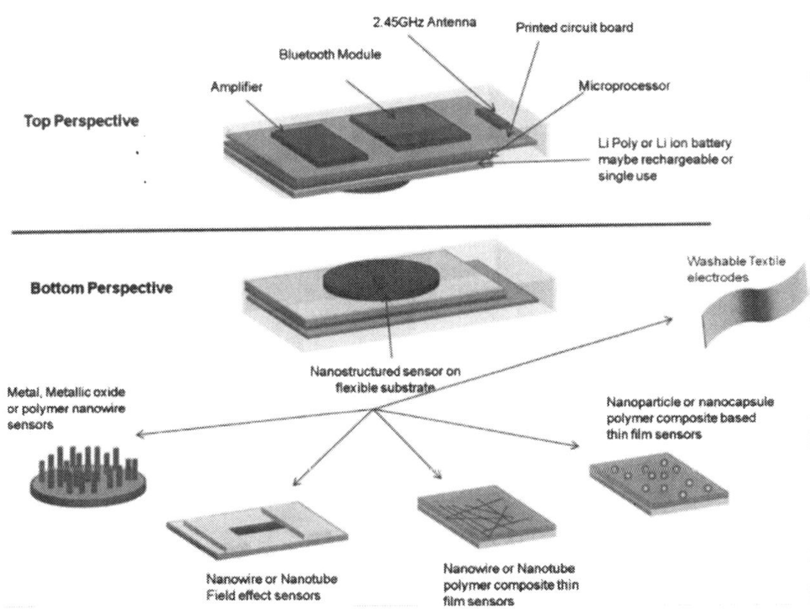

Figure 3-3 Top and bottom perspectives of the e-Nanoflex system.

microcontroller for converting the analog output of the amplifier into a stream of digitized numbers, and the Bluetooth radio module for transmitting the acquired data are combined into a single, double-sided printed circuit board (PCB) module. The stacking of various components combined with nanostructured sensors results in a small form factor that can be used for various wireless sensor applications involving physiological health monitoring. Flexible thin film sensors for many biological parameters, such as an organic light emitting diode (OLED) and an organic photodiode (OPD) based pulse oximetry, a polymeric piezoelectric based sensor for respiratory air flow and respiration effort, and a flexible electrode for bioelectrical signals, such as ECG, EMG, EOG, and EEG, can be interfaced with the e-Nanoflex system.

3.5.2 Data transfer and backend storage

Figure 3-4 schematically presents the data flow in the e-nanoflex system. The sensor and the amplifier constitute the analog front end. The signals obtained from the sensors are usually weak and noise inflicted. For example, 60 Hz interference noise is common in the acquired electrical signals. The amplifier and filter circuits determine the quality of the signals obtained by the sensor, so they play a vital role in maintaining the integrity of the

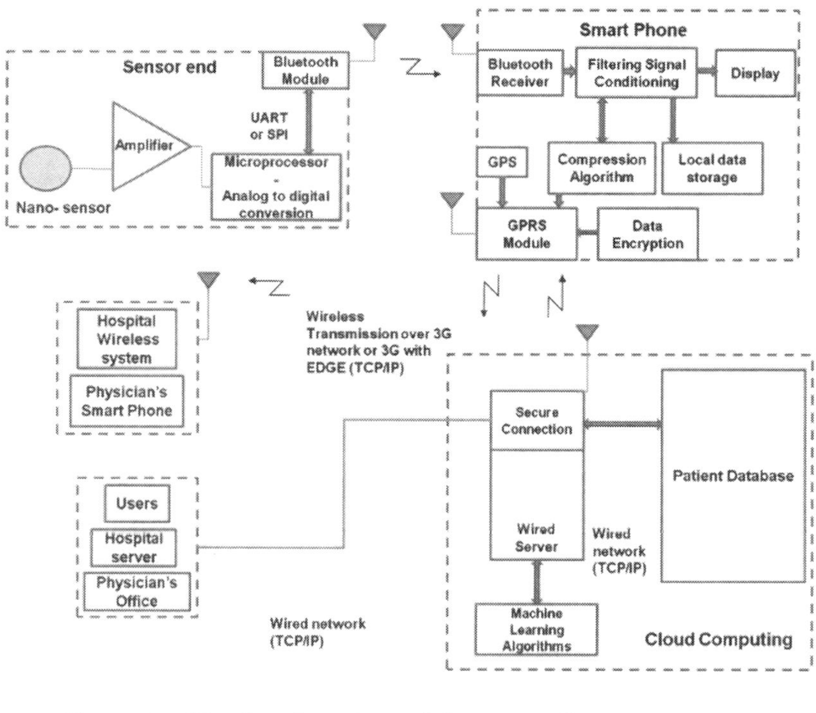

Figure 3-4 The data flow chart of the e-Nanoflex system.

biosignals. The amplifier output is then digitized by a microcontroller. The microcontroller is used to fix the sampling rate of the ADC. The data processed by the microcontroller is presented as a string of digital numbers ready to be transferred to the Smartphone. The Smartphone first scans for the e-Nanoflex sensor system and establishes a secure connection through a 16 character pin code for device pairing. Once a connection is established with the e-Nanoflex system, the microcontroller on the sensor end starts relaying the data from ADC outputs to the Bluetooth module.

The data from the e-Nanoflex sensors are received by the Smartphone, which act as a base station from which the data are relayed to a remote server. As implementing computationally intensive abnormality-detection services locally on a Smartphone can be a huge energy and CPU drain, e-Nanoflex provides a partitioned approach, where computation is divided into two components: the low overhead simple computation on the local Smartphone device, and the intensive abnormality analysis and adaptive filtering at the backend. Such an intelligent division of computation between the Smartphone and the backend cloud provides several advantages. First, the system is germane to the resource constraints on the mobile device. Second, it makes complex adaptive filtering, mandatory to the removal of motion artifacts, possible at the backend cloud.

3.5.3 Data processing and relaying by Smartphone

As almost all the Smartphones are Bluetooth-enabled, Bluetooth is used as the radio for data communication between the sensor module and the Smartphone. The data received from the sensor using the Bluetooth module need filtering since several motion artifacts cannot be effectively removed by the hardware. To ameliorate this issue, the Smartphone runs simple filtering algorithms. Note that computationally intensive filtering schemes are executed on the cloud since the mobile device lacks the computing capability to execute such algorithms. The filtering process on the phone uses simple digital filters, implemented as linear difference equations. This signal is then stored on the local storage device or displayed upon request by the user. The data are then relayed to a backend cloud service using http over a 3G or WiFi connection.

The data are sampled and transferred at a frequency in the order of hundreds of Hertz. For example, for ECG, the sampling rate is 200 Hz. If the data in their raw form are relayed to the backend cloud, it can potentially choke the cellular channel. Currently available 3G networks cannot support such high volumes of communication at all times due to channel sharing. Therefore, data compression algorithms are required to keep the amount of data to a minimum. Data from biomedical sensors, such as ECG, are periodic and predictable and hence e-Nanoflex uses a simple differencing based algorithm, followed by entropy based compression techniques, to minimize the data to be transmitted. The data transmitted to the remote server are geo-tagged. The onboard global positioning system (GPS) on a Smartphone provides the current latitude and longitude of the patient. At the remote server end, e-Nanoplast stores the geo-tagged sensor data in a secure database.

3.5.4 Data security considerations

Since the e-Nanoflex platform continuously streams critical healthcare data to a backend database, security and data integrity are critical for maintaining patient data confidentiality. The data transfer channel between the sensor and the Smartphone as well as the backend cloud is susceptible to pernicious security attacks. For instance, the e-Nanoflex sensor wireless channel is susceptible to "sniffing attacks", where a malicious entity can tap into the channel and access the data using a tuned off-the-shelf software radio. Once the information is extracted, the captured data can be placed back on the network or replayed. Additionally, battery powered devices are vulnerable to Denial of Service (DoS) attacks, where legitimate users are denied to access the remote server by malicious programs that block service, and battery-drain attacks, wherein a malicious user pretends to be a sensor and continuously sends data to the Smartphone and drains its battery. Further, data stored at the back-end databases should be accessible to authorized hospitals and physicians only.

In the e-Nanoflex system, the data security is achieved mainly by three approaches. First, sniffing attacks are tackled by using standard data encryption over Bluetooth. Secondly, DoS attacks are avoided using power analysis. Finally, at the backend, standard authentication measures are implemented on web servers to assure that the data communication link between the caregivers and the backend database is secure.

3.5.5 Cloud services

Once the data are offloaded to a remote server, they are stored in a large scale patient centric secure database. In anticipation of large scale deployment of e-Nanoflex sensor systems with continuous monitoring, the sheer volume of data will require automated signal analysis and anomaly detection techniques. Therefore, e-Nanoflex implements machine learning algorithms, such as discriminant analysis, to extract features from the collected data. The type of features depends on the disease class being studied, for example, simple features, such as the empirical mean, are sufficient for diabetes but more complex features, such as interwave width, are required for heart disease analysis. These features can be used to detect abnormalities in the data collected. The cloud services, upon determining a state of emergency, can send an alert message in the form of a short messaging service (SMS) or a multimedia message with an image of the abnormal data and the location of the patient to the attending physician's Smartphone. An SMS can also be sent to the nearest emergency medical service team, based on the current location from GPS reading.

4. Smart textile based wearable health monitoring systems

This chapter discusses the development of smart textile based wearable health monitoring systems (ST-WHMSs). After introducing the concepts of smart textiles and printable electronics, textile sensor technology is discussed, followed by the roll-to-roll fabrication techniques, which can be used for mass fabrication of low-cost ST-WHMSs.

4.1 Smart textiles

The primary motivation for, and the main purpose of, the development of ST-WHMSs is to enhance the quality of life for individuals. ST-WHMSs are a natural interface for the end users, offering a sense of security while not being perceived as a medical device [21]. They provide an elegant solution to the requirements of individuals across a wide range of ages. They can be used to monitor young or elderly recuperating/convalescent patients either in hospital or at home, and they can also be used by athletes to monitor important physiological parameters so that their training or fitness program can be improved in a timely fashion.

ST-WHMHSs are available in a variety of ways, i.e: vests, bed sheets, pillow covers and caps. Textiles offer a durable platform for embedded sensors and communication systems, with the components stitched or woven into the fabric or attached to it in form of sensor and communication chipsets. Individual electronics can be mounted on the textile and connected through wires that have been built in or manufactured in the textile itself. Both durable and removable sensors and communication electronics can be incorporated in smart textile products. In the development of smart textile products, it should be kept in mind that the final product should still be wearable, comfortable and washable. Therefore, the embedment of the electronic functionality should not sacrifice the textile properties of the products.

Yarns play an important role in the development of smart textiles and ST-WHMSs [4, 42]. Yarns should have desirable electrical, electronic, mechanical, and electrochemical properties. Conductive yarns can be polyamide coated with a thin layer of silver on which other metals, such as Au and Pt, are galvanically deposited. Conductive yarns can also be made of silver or copper threads twisted with natural or artificial fibers. All these conductive yarns can be sewn, embroidered, knitted, and woven using standard machines because of their elastic properties.

There are two important impediments to the development of ST-WHMSs. The first is the seamless integration of flexible electrodes, flexible sensors, signal conditioning circuits and data logging or wireless transmission devices into a garment. The second is the low-cost mass-manufacture method. Roll-to-roll printing and screen printing are two low-cost methods for mass manufacture on flexible substrates and can be extended to textiles as well. More discussions about roll-to-roll manufacturing occur in Section 4.4.

4.2 Printable electronics

Printing technologies have been well established for making complex high resolution designs on a wide range of substrates, including textiles. Recently, the same attributes have been demonstrated for printed electronics. Printing allows for direct pattern transfer of electronics using lesser materials and creating no or little waste, which is a better alternative to photolithography techniques. Among the popular printing technologies, screen printing and gravure printing are well suited for mass fabrication of electronics on textiles because they are a parallel printing technology. The attribute of parallel printing, as compared to serial printing technologies like ink jet printing, helps to increase throughput towards low cost production. These technologies enable fabrication (over a large surface area) of electronics with varied functionality: sensor systems and flexible printed circuits for embedded wireless telemetry systems. Flexible substrates like polyimide (Kapton), Mylar, Polyethylenenapthalate (PEN), PET have been used for the fabrication of printed electronics, and similar processes can be accomplished on fabric substrates. These sensor systems can be incorporated (enmeshed) in textile fabrics or the sensor patterns can be made on the textile itself. Though the printing processes can produce conductive traces with thickness down to about 100 μm, the traces on a fabric may be required to be thicker in order to avoid the disruption due to stretching of the fabric.

As shown in Figure 4-1, sensors can be mass produced, as an array of devices, on a flexible substrate, and traces for electronic circuitry can be

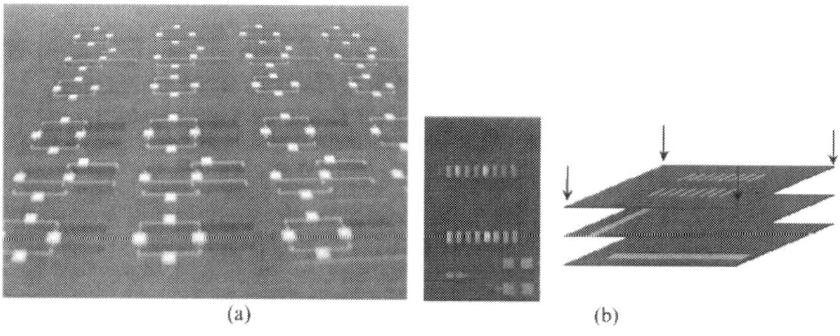

Figure 4-1 (a) Array of sensors printed on polyimide substrate, (b) Flexible printed circuit for mounting silicon based components.

printed and laminated to obtain printed circuit flexible boards. Therefore, sensors and amplifier-transmitter components can be accommodated on or enmeshed in fabric or other flexible substrates. It is important that the electro-opto-mechanical functionalities should be incorporated in the textile while keeping the textile properties of the product (system). To achieve cost effective manufacturing, in the choice of screen printing and gravure printing technologies, it should be ensured that the fabrication process shall not deviate significantly from garment making techniques [7].

4.3 Textile sensor technology

Physiological signals, such as ECG, pulse rate, body temperature, respiratory effort and blood pressure, provide a comprehensive medical status of a person. In the following, textile sensor technologies for monitoring these physiological signals will be discussed.

4.3.1 Electrocardiogram (ECG)

An ECG sensor system is basically a set of electrodes for detecting the electric pulse traveling through the skin due to the depolarization of cardiac muscle cells. A basic ECG set up consists of at least three electrodes, and they are used in pairs, known as leads, to record the ECG signals. Conventional ECG recording is done with the help of silver/silver chloride electrodes with conductive gel for contact with skin. Figure 4-2 (a) shows metal coated nylon electrodes, and in ECG measurements, they are in contact with skin without any gel. ECG signals are the potential across the load resistance between the two electrodes that can be conceived as the impedance due to body bulk, skin and electrodes, as shown in Figure 4-2 (b). These electrodes are required to be big enough, 1"×3" in this case, for consistency of contact with the skin. The wearable dry electrode technology works as well as the wet electrode technology, and it is good for long term monitoring as no gel is needed.

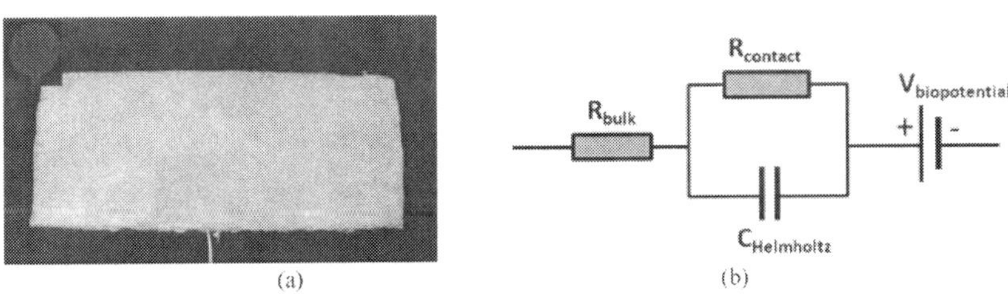

(a) (b)

Figure 4-2 (a) Metal coated fiber dry electrode that is integrable in a textile platform, (b) Equivalent circuit model for dry electrode-skin interface.

4.3.2 Pulse rate

The pulse rate sensor system is a real time signal analyzer that detects the R (ventricular depolarization) peak in the ECG signal. The R peak represents the contraction of the left ventricle i.e. pumping of the blood to the aorta (the main artery). Though the entire ECG signature of P, Q, R, S and T waves is representative of heartbeats, the R peaks are the highest and easy to detect. By using the Pan and Tompkins algorithm [43], a robust frequency based peak sorting algorithm, the number of R peaks per minute can be calculated, and the time interval between two consecutive R peak (R-R interval) can be profiled as heart rate variability in time and frequency domains for diagnosis.

4.3.3 Temperature monitoring

The temperature sensing system is a resistive temperature detector (RTD) element arranged as one of the resistive elements in a Wheatstone Bridge configuration, as shown in Figure 4-3 (a). The RTD element was a conducting channel that has a high width to length ratio for improved heat exchange. The conductive material was carbon black based conductive paste with high thermal coefficient for resistance. The other three resistive elements of the bridge were made of the same conductive paste but were encapsulated in an electrically insulating heat sealant. The silver ink based conductive lines have a very low thermal coefficient for resistance and were used for electrical connections. The output voltage was measured with a constant input voltage and varying temperature, from which the RTD resistance was derived and calibrated against temperature. The temperature sensor was mounted against the axillary auxiliary site of the arm, as shown in Figure 4-3 (c). The axillary body temperature is considered as a surrogate for the oral or rectal body temperature as it is convenient for subjects especially young children.

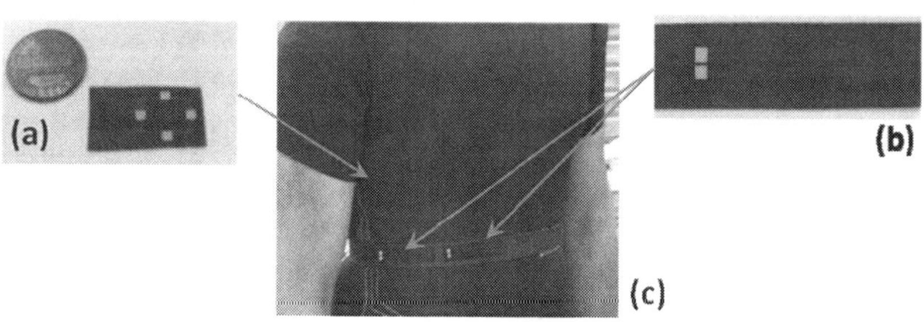

Figure 4-3 (a) resistive temperature detector based temperature sensor element, (b) strain sensitive element for abdominal respiration effort sensor, (c) textile based platform with the temperature and respiration sensors mounted on the axillary region of the arm and the upper abdomen, respectively.

4.3.4 Respiration effort

The respiration effort sensor system is a strain sensitive element incorporated in a Wheatstone bridge configuration, as a strain gauge, as shown in Figure 4-3 (b). The strain sensitive element was a conducting channel that has a low width to length ratio and aligned along the axis of strain for improved strain profiling. The conductive material was carbon black based conductive paste with high linear elastic coefficient of resistance. The other three resistive elements of the bridge were made of the same conductive paste but were mounted traverse to the strain axis. All the resistive components were capsulated in an electrically insulating heat sealant. The silver ink based conductive lines had a very low linear elastic coefficient of resistance and were used for electrical connections. The strain gauge setup was on the upper abdomen region for measuring the abdominal distention, as shown in Figure 4-3 (c). The signal can be used to estimate the frequency and amplitude of respiration effort relative to basal respiration effort.

4.3.5 Blood pressure

In this method, the pulse transit time is measured for estimation of arterial blood pressure. As discussed in Section 2.4, a beat by beat monitoring system can be used for blood pressure test. An infrared reflectance based photoplethysmography device is mounted on the arm to monitor pulse waves in the brachial artery [44]. It measures the reflectance of infrared by the blood flowing in the brachial artery. Therefore, the pulse waves in the blood flow can be measured as the reflectance profile detected by the device. The ventricular discharge (R peak) is registered as pulse wave initiation and the lagging pulse wave measured at the brachial artery site is the culmination point. Hence, the pulse transit time in the left arm brachial artery was measured, and the blood pressure can be estimated by Eq. (2).

4.3.6 Typical results

The sensor systems were mounted on a wearable textile based platform. The monitoring sites for sensors were identified for testing: (i) right arm, left arm and left leg for ECG, (ii) axillary site of the arm for body temperature, (iii) upper abdomen for respiration effort, and (iv) brachial artery for pulse wave. The sensors were accordingly integrated or enmeshed in the textile by tacking them with threads and needles, and drawing out connections using metal coated nylon threads. To maintain the ergonomics of the sensor systems, the skin of the subject was not prepped in any way. A real time signal acquisition system was set up to acquire five sensor signals and plot them on a remote computation device.

The ECG dry electrode sensor system was tested against the standard silver/silver chloride wet electrodes for signal quality. As shown in Figure 4-4, two Lead II (right arm-left leg) ECG Signals were acquired and compared. With reference to the standard electrodes, the base line of the dry electrode ECG signal was stable but with a hint of respiration artifact. The respiration

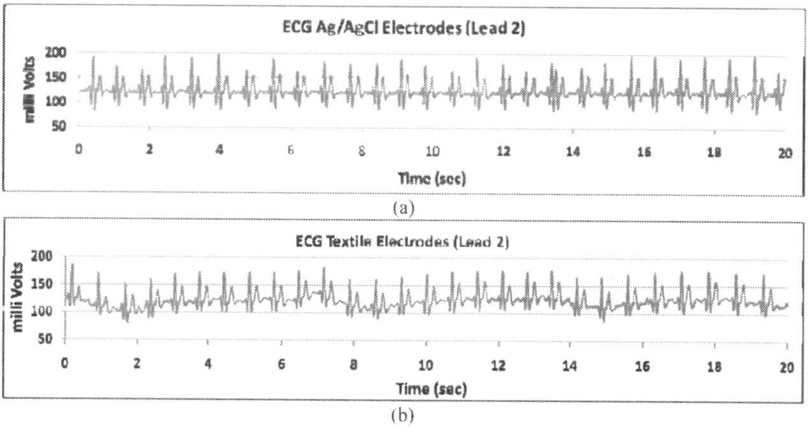

Figure 4-4 Lead II electrocardiograph signals from different electrodes. (a) Silver-silver chloride wet/gel electrodes, (b) metal coated textile dry electrodes.

artifacts can be attributed to triboelectric noises introduced through the fabric based connections between the electrodes and the amplifier-transmitter module. The peak to peak amplitude was consistent and comparable to the standard. The constituent P, Q, R, S and T waveforms were visible in the dry electrodes' signal. Therefore the signal from the dry electrodes can be used for diagnostic purposes, such as heart rate variability and waveform intervals.

The respiration sensor was mounted on the upper abdomen to detect the distention of the thoracic cavity due to respiration intake. The subject was asked to do a sequence of normal breathing, deep breath and fast breathing. The signal acquired was plotted as the output voltage of the amplifier. The amplitude and frequency of respiration effort for each segment were shown in Figure 4-5 (a), (b), and (c) respectively. The signals clearly indicated the respiratory cycles.

The calibration for the RTD sensor system was carried out on a thermally isolated hot surface with a temperature control. The temperature sensor signals were amplified and transmitted as the output voltage from the voltage divider circuit. The signal was used to derive the resistance of the RTD element and plotted against the surface temperature. The calibration curve was obtained by polynomial curve fitting as shown in Figure 4-6. The sensor response shows saturation at temperatures in excess of 40 °C. The range of linear response is 32 °C to 38 °C, which is the range of axillary temperature that covers from normal condition to feverish [45].

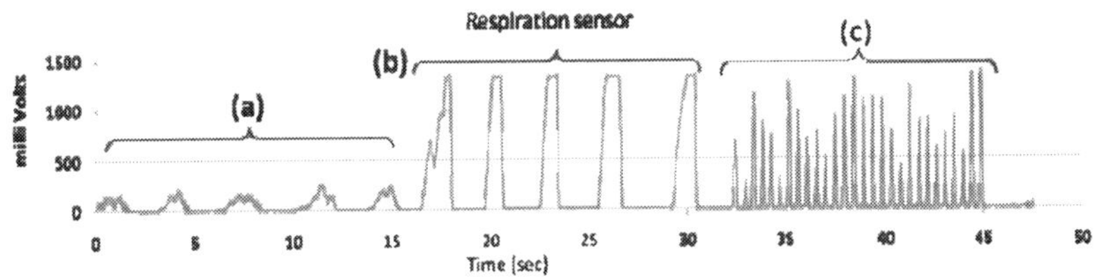

Figure 4-5 Respiration effort data showing frequency and inhalation peak upon (a) normal breathing, (b) deep breathing, (c) fast breathing.

Real-time signals from the Lead II ECG (between Right Arm and Left Leg limb electrodes) sensor and the photoplethysmography device at the brachial artery site were acquired. As shown in Figure 4-7, the signals exhibit a measurable time lag that is the transit time from the ventricular discharge to the brachial artery site. The Pan and Tompkins peak sorting algorithm is capable of sorting R peaks and the pulse peaks for estimating the pulse transit time and deriving the arterial blood pressure.

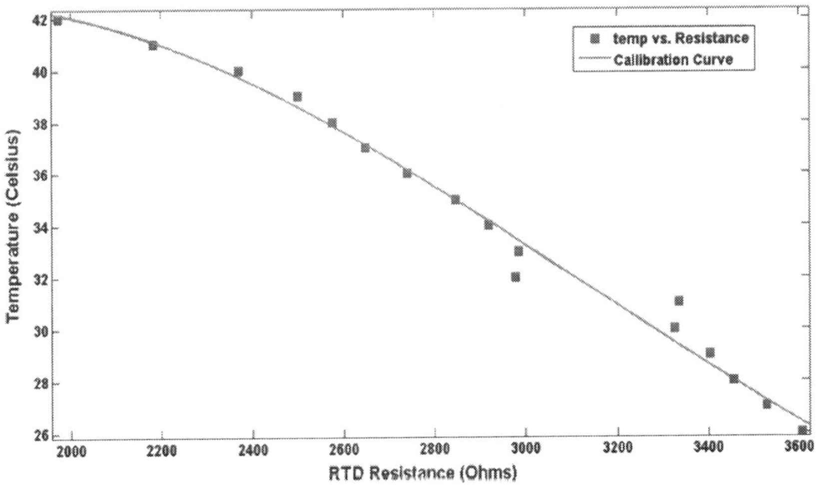

Figure 4-6 Resistive Temperature Detector based temperature sensor calibration curve: Temperature (°C) vs. Resistance (Ω). The calibration curve is given by the equation $T = (2.07\times10^{-9}) r^3 - (1.93\times10^{-5})r^2 + 0.0485r + 5.72$, and R^2 value for the curve fitting is 0.988.

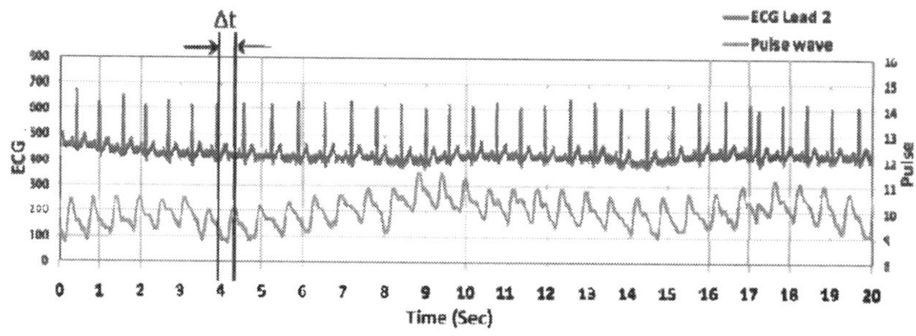

Figure 4-7 Leading electrocardiograph (Lead II) and lagging brachial artery pulse data acquired on the same time line for measurement of pulse transit time (Δt).

4.4 Roll-to-roll fabrication techniques

Roll-to-roll fabrication techniques shall enable economic production of the consumable components for mobile wearable health monitoring systems [18]. In the following, the state-of-the-art gravure printing and solution based electrochemical nanowire array synthesis are discussed for the fabrication of mobile wearable nano-bio health monitoring systems.

Gravure printing is an alternative to the widely used PCB technology. It incorporates printed circuit layouts to flexible films in roll-to-roll

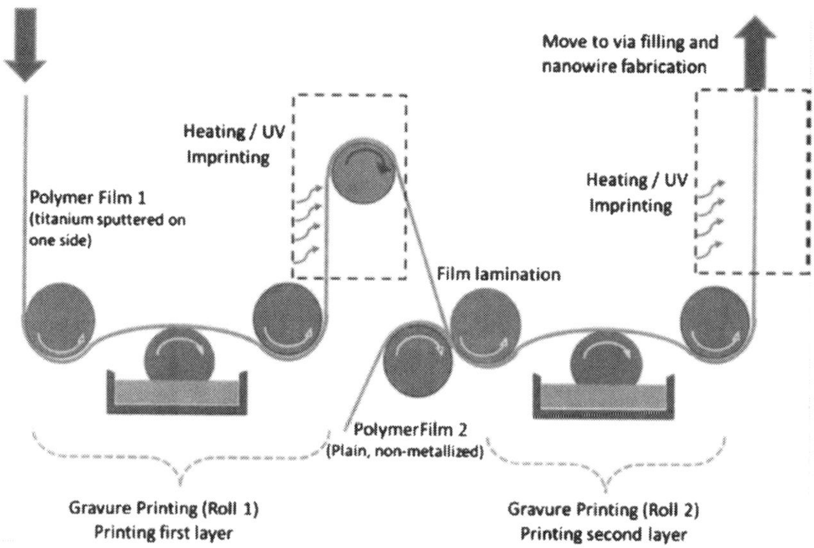

Figure 4-8 Roll to roll fabrication for printed circuit flexible platform.

manufacturing. The circuit layouts can be printed on different flexible films, laminated and interconnected, to construct a multilayer flexible printed circuit platform, as shown in Figure 4-8. The lamination process involves punching via lines for interlayer connections, alignment, lamination, and via filling.

For nanowire synthesis, the laminated flexible platform is coated with resist polymer on the titanium coated face. As shown in Figure 4-9, the film roll is moved to the nano-imprint drum. The drum is mounted with a metallic nano-imprint stamp. The polymer film is patterned and cured to obtain a template with nanoscale pores. The roll proceeds to an electrolyte tank for gold deposition. This process takes 15–30 min, and during this period, the roll conveyor is stopped. After that, the roll is moved and the process is repeated for the next portion of the roll.

The large-scale and high-throughput manufacturing of such a system plays a key role in keeping the final cost for the end user low. For ECG monitoring, the gold nanowire is made on flexible metal foil substrates and is thus compatible with production techniques such as roll-to-roll manufacturing. Printed circuit traces on flexible substrates have recently emerged on flexible substrates such as polyimide, and they are also compatible with roll-to-roll manufacturing technology.

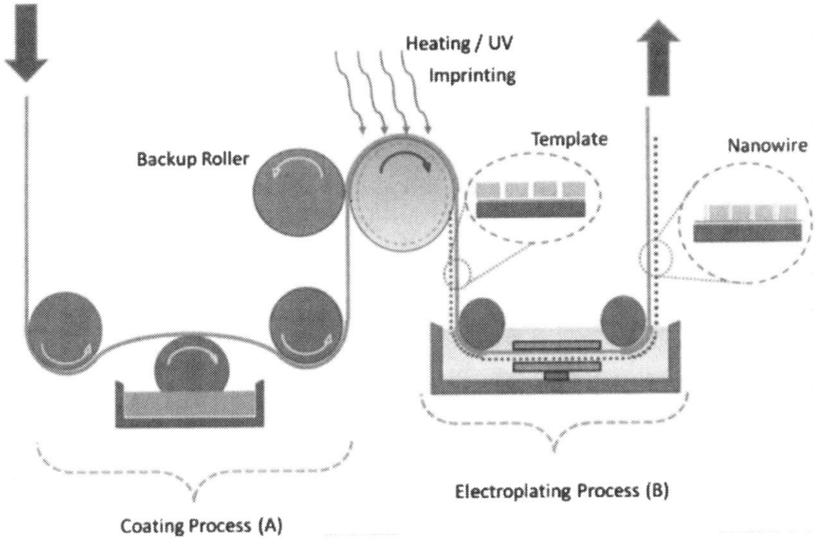

Figure 4-9 Roll to roll fabrication for nanowire electrodes.

5. Case studies

In this chapter, four case studies on the applications of mobile wearable health monitoring systems are discussed. The systems in these cases have the same or similar wireless communication and data storage sub-systems. As different sensors are used, they have different medical functionalities.

5.1 Cardiac health monitoring

The e-Nanoflex with gold nanowire electrodes was used to acquire ECG signals. ECG is the first diagnostic test carried out by a cardiac physician to diagnose cardiac ailments. Many health parameters can be derived from ECG signals. For example, the inverse of the interval between two consecutive R peaks of the ECG waveform provides the heart rate. Another salient feature of this ECG case study is the use of dry electrodes. Gold nano-electrodes do not require any gel and can acquire signals through hair without the need to clean the skin with alcohol swabs. These electrodes also have an unlimited shelf-life and are reusable after sterilization because of the inert nature of gold. Therefore, the e-Nanoflex system with dry gold nanoelectrodes is ideally suited for minimally intrusive ECG monitoring.

Nanowire electrodes were fabricated on a flexible titanium foil. Figure 5-1 (a) shows a scanning electron microscope image of the nanowire structures on the electrodes, and Figure 5-1 (b) shows how the electrodes were mounted on a standard medical plaster for superficial wound dressing. The nanowires have an average height of about 1 μm.

The three limb lead signals were obtained from commercial wet Ag/AgCl electrodes (Moore Medical LLC, Farmington, CT) and from gold nanowire electrodes, respectively, as shown in Figure 5-2 [18]. The signals from the two types of electrodes are observably similar. The data from the e-Nanoflex sensors were sent to a remote server through the 3G network. The data were tagged with the current GPS location and the time. In case of an emergency, a message with recorded data and current location and time can be sent to the emergency response team.

5.2 e-bra for ECG measurement for women

An e-bra is a platform on which various sensors for cardiac health monitoring can be integrated into the fabric [40]. It is an autonomous garment that can collect and transmit vital health signals from the wearer to any desired location through connections to a Smartphone and the cellular network or through a Bluetooth enabled PC and the Internet.

Mortality due to cardiac related ailments has been consistently higher in women as compared with men in the United States. Gender related differences in specificity of regular noninvasive diagnostic tools and the lack of a clear understanding of the effect of postmenopausal hormonal changes in

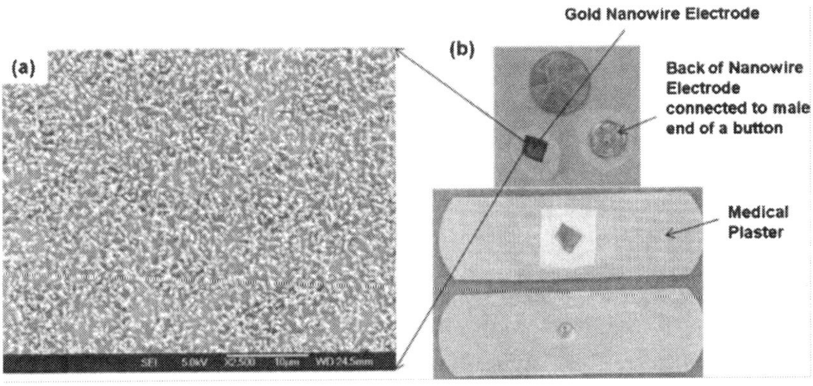

Figure 5-1 (a) Scanning electron microscope image of vertical gold nanowires. (b) The gold nanowire electrode packaged in a medical plaster.

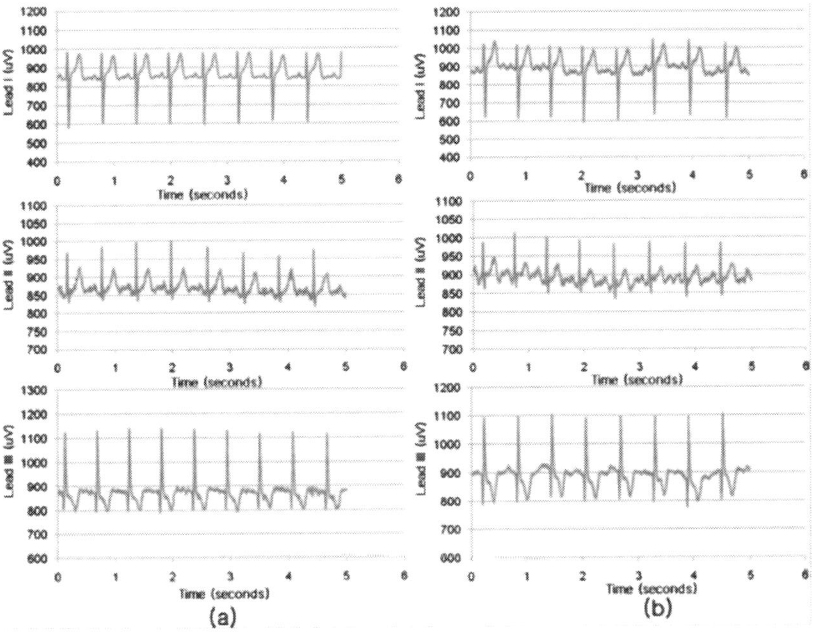

Figure 5-2 Three limb lead ECGs acquired from e-Nanoflex sensor using (a) commercial Ag/AgCl electrodes and (b) gold nanowire electrodes.

women have been cited as the two main reasons for this disparity. Recent advances in secondary and tertiary diagnostic information extraction techniques from signals such as ECG through HRV analysis and wavelet domain analysis techniques have revealed many differences in autonomic nervous-cardiovascular activity regulation, between men and women. At this stage, disease management may be the only option as opposed to preventive treatments, and continuous and long-term monitoring is an essential requirement.

An e-bra platform for nanosensors can be used for seamless cardiovascular monitoring. The sensors, nanomaterial or textile based dry electrodes, acquire the electrocardiograph signals, which are sent to a textile mounted wireless module. A Smartphone or a wireless Bluetooth enabled PC receives these data and stores or processes the information when necessary. The use of a Smartphone as a base station for receiving data offers the advantage of cellular network connectivity to the Internet and consequently cloud computing resources for more complex computations such as feature extraction and automatic diagnosis.

Figure 5-3 (a) shows the electrode placements for a 12-lead system and Figure 5-3 (b) shows a similar implementation on an e-bra with textiles or gold nanowire electrodes. Figure 5-4 (a) shows a picture of an e-bra and an e-Nanoflex module used for data acquisition and wireless transmission.

ECG data were acquired from two subjects with the e-bra. Commercially available electrodes for ECG are usually Ag/AgCl electrodes with a conductive gel that minimizes the impedance between the skin and the electrode. Dry electrodes offer a much more comfortable and durable alternative. To develop a garment needs that can pick up good quality ECG and be worn everyday and throughout the day, it is necessary to use dry and washable

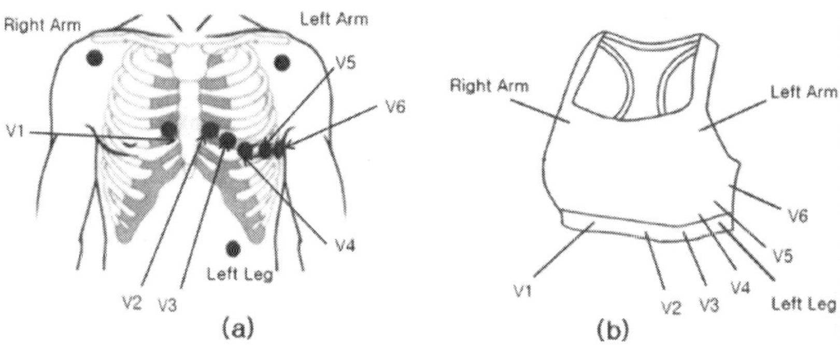

Figure 5-3 (a) Lead placement for 12 lead ECG with derived limb leads and (b) similar placement on the e-bra.

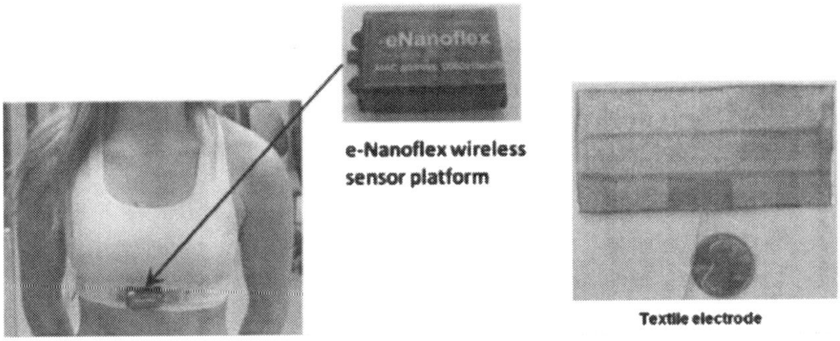

Figure 5-4 (a) An e-bra with an e-Nanoflex module, worn by one of the test subjects. (b) Conductive fabric electrodes in the e-bra.

electrodes such as gold nanowire electrodes or conductive fabric based electrodes that can be easily stitched onto the e-bra.

Figure 5-4 (b) shows a conductive fabric electrode that can be used for acquiring ECG signals. For ECG monitoring with the e-bra, two such electrodes were placed in the positions described as V_1 and V_2, as shown in Figure 5-5 (a). The potential difference between these two positions shows

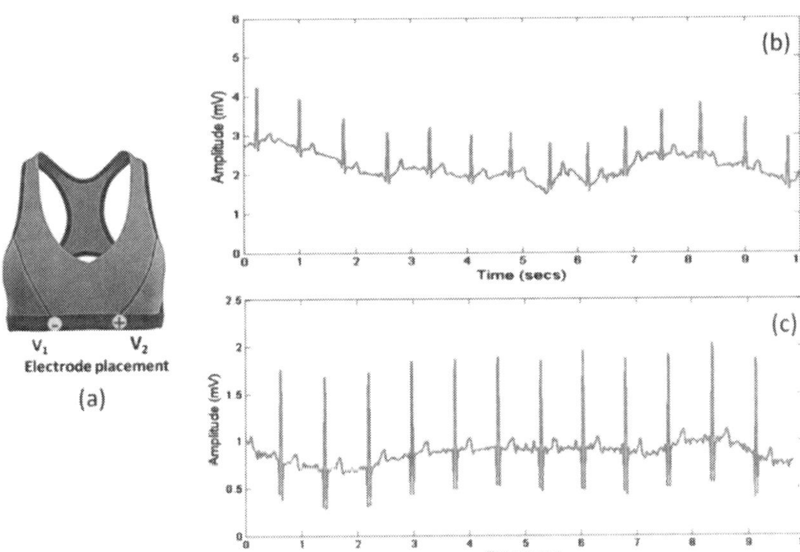

Figure 5-5 (a) The electrode positions on the e-bra, (b) data acquired from subject 1, and (c) data acquired from subject 2.

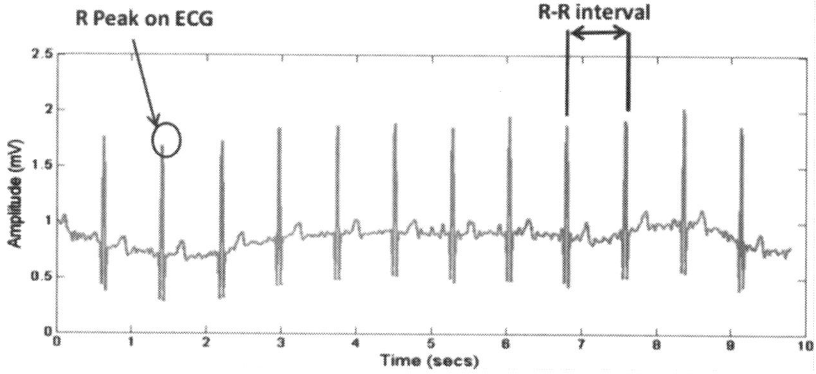

Figure 5-6 R-R interval determination from ECG.

a distinct and sharp peak in the signal that corresponds to the activation of the left ventricle of the heart, namely, the R peak of the ECG. The signal also shows Q, S, and T waveforms, where the S-T segment is related to the ventricular repolarization. Figures 5-5(b) and 5-5(c) show the data acquired from two healthy subjects, respectively [40].

Heart rate variability analysis is an important prognostic and diagnostic technique. Heart rate variability is the sequence formed by concatenating the difference in heart rate between consecutive beats. The inverse of this quantity is the difference in the intervals between consecutive R peaks. By detecting the R peaks, the interval between them and hence the heart rate variability signal against beats can be obtained, as shown in Figure 5-6.

The autoregressive (AR) power spectrum estimation technique was used to obtain the power spectrum density (PSD) plot with the characteristic

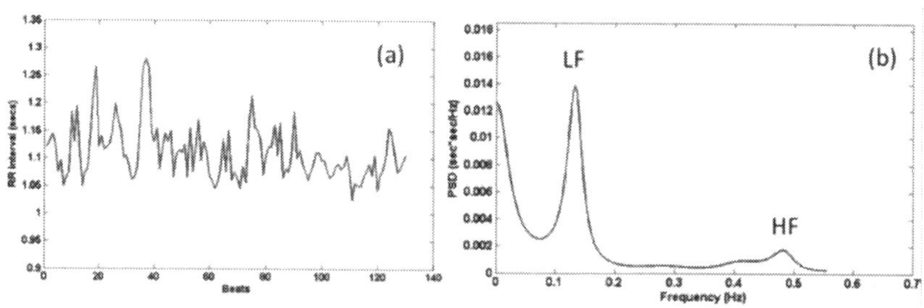

Figure 5-7 (a) Plot of the RR interval series against beat number and (b) plot of the AR PSD computed from the RRI series for the standing case.

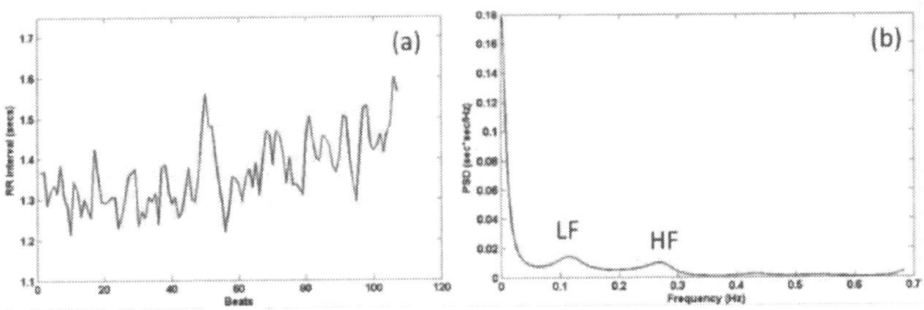

Figure 5-8 (a) Plot of the RR interval series against beat number and (b) plot of the AR PSD computed from the RRI series for the head-up tilt with a supine position.

LF and HF peaks [46]. The AR PSD is ideal for short data record lengths and performs very well as a frequency estimator for signals with strong sinusoidal components such as HRV signals. ECG data (150 seconds) were collected for a healthy female of age 18 in a supine position and in a standing still state, respectively. Figure 5-7 shows the RR interval series plotted against beats and the AR PSD computed from the RRI series for the standing case. Figure 5-8 shows the same for a supine ECG. In the case of head-up tilt, the heart rate was higher as compared with the supine ECG. The classic shift in the power distribution between LF and HF components with respect to the total power in each case is evident from the AR PSDs in Figures 5-7 (b) and 5-8 (b). Thus, the e-bra is a reliable system for tracking chronic conditions related to the autonomous nervous regulation of cardiac activity.

5.3 Smart vest for ECG and blood pressure measurement for men

This cardiac health monitoring system works on the principle of unhindered-pervasive physiological sensing, in proximity or in contact with the body. The prototype system is a body conforming inner vest [36]. It has textile based or integrated sensors for multi-lead ECG, heart rate variability and blood pressure sensing, and wireless communication, as shown in Figure 5-9.

The instrumentation of the textile based or textile integrable sensor system was designed for seamless integration in the textile. The electronic connections, for relaying signals and supplying power to the sensor modules, were made out of conductive thread with tribo-electric resistant insulation. The ECG electrodes were mounted with connections made by conductive yarns. The PPG band for blood pressure monitoring, with infrared emitter-detector arrays, was worn separately and connected to the conductive thread lines on the vest for signal relay as shown in Figure 5-9.

Signals from the sensors were routed to a signal conditioning and wireless data transmission module. This module was fashioned like a small card

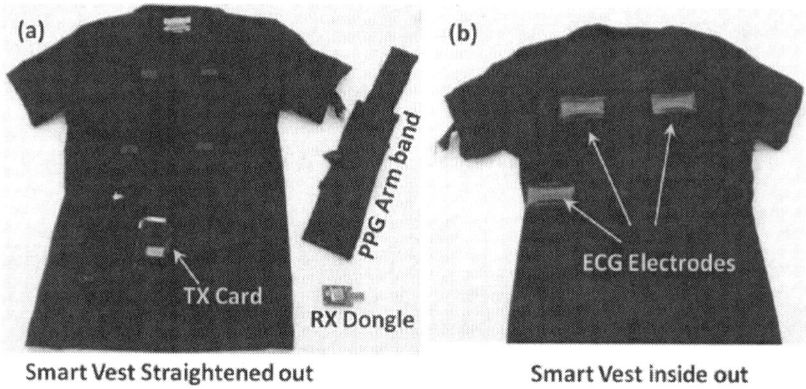

Figure 5-9 Smart healthcare textile system showing (a) transmitter (TX) card, receiver (RX) dongle and plethysmograph (PPG) arm band, and (b) ECG electrodes.

so that it can be easily slipped into a pocket on the vest, allowing for the vest to be an autonomous sensing platform. The block diagram of the card circuit is shown below in Figure 5-10. In combination with a laptop computer for wireless data reception, the smart vest was tested as a mobile wearable health monitoring system.

5.3.1 Electrocardiograph (ECG) and heart rate

ECGs are the procedure of first choice in the evaluation of patients with chest pain, syncope, or dizziness. They are also used as a baseline test, for evaluation of response to therapy, for follow-up, and before surgery [47]. As shown in Figure 2-2 (a), a three electrode system is often used to record

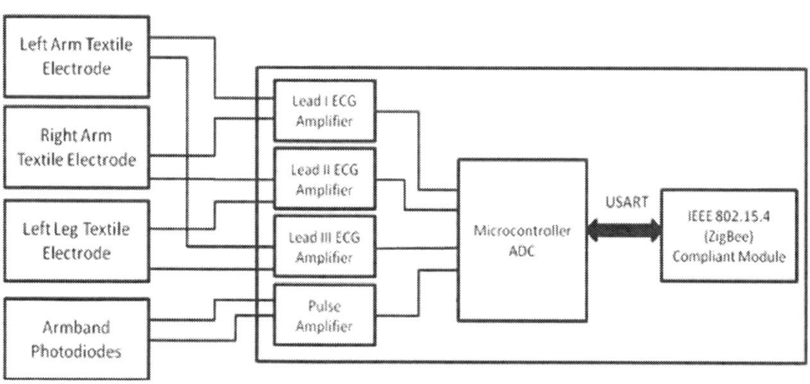

Figure 5-10 Block diagram of the transmission module for a multi parameter health monitoring smart textile.

ECG signals. The electrodes in a three electrode system are augmented right arm (RA), left arm (LA) and left leg (LL), and they are used in pairs or leads. The electrodes used for this smart textile system were dry metalized fabric based electrodes, as an alternative to conventional conductive gel based silver/silver chloride wet electrodes. The ECG signal obtained from this system was compared with the ECG readout from standard cardiograph as shown in Figure 5-11. The heart rate can be derived through a real time signal processing application, which is based on the Pan and Tompkins algorithm for R peak detection.

The subjects for this study were adult males between age of 25 and 60 years. The subjects were asked to put on the smart healthcare textile (vest) system and data were recorded for 30 minutes. The heights and arm spans of the subjects were recorded for blood pressure calibration. The ECG signals were acquired in real time and processed through a band pass filter to remove

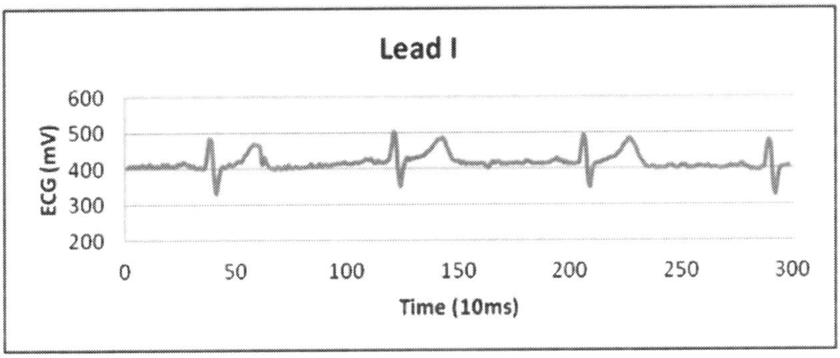

(a)

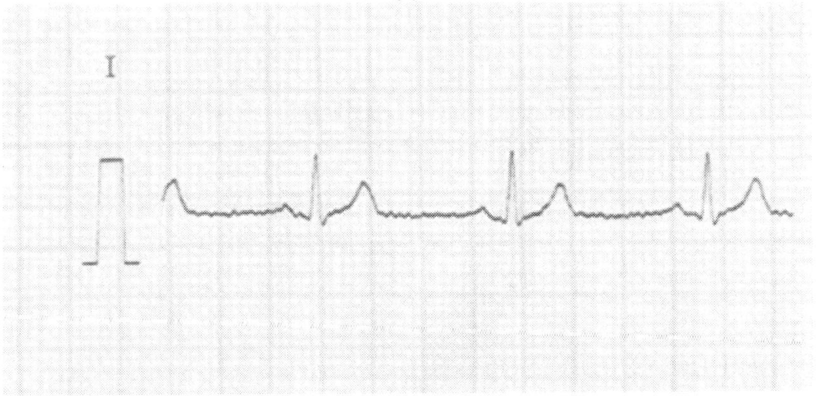

(b)

Figure 5-11 ECG Waveform comparison. (a) Lead I ECG from the smart healthcare textile system. (b) Lead I ECG readout from a standard cardiogram equipment.

any residual 60 Hz noise. Augmented Lead I ECG signals were compared with the standard limb Lead I ECG signals. It was found that while Q and T waveforms matched for all the subjects, and R and S waveforms were similar for half of the subjects. This was mainly because textile system R waves were of lower amplitude as compared to those in standard signals and the S wave notches were deeper than those in standard signals. The QRS complexes were similar. A similar trend was observed in case of P waves, which was because of the P waves not being visible over the baseline. These dissimilarities can be attributed to variation of the augmented RA and LA electrodes. Every subject, by virtue of his shoulder size, fits differently into vests (general sizes small, medium and large). Due to this, the RA and LA electrodes are not necessarily placed between first two ribs below collar bone (clavicle) on right and left side of the chest respectively. However, the R and S amplitude variance should not affect their diagnostic value in calculation of time stamps such as QT interval, ST segment and QRS complex width. Similarly, the P waves become more profound when the electrodes RA and LA are placed at their respective positions above atrial plane of the heart [30].

The signals from Lead II ECG were of better match. This can be attributed to the placement of the RA and LL electrodes, which is always across the left ventricle. The signals from Lead III ECG showed some dissimilarity because of the variance in the position of electrode LA. The Lead III signal also showed ambiguity mostly in the Q, R, and S magnitudes. The magnitude of the QRS complex is important for determining the cardiac vector and can be determined from Leads I and II that conform well to the standard. Therefore, the collective data from three augmented limb leads can be used for medical diagnosis.

5.3.2 Cuff less blood pressure measurement

A textile mounted infrared system that is a modified form of photoplethysmography (PPG) system was used to monitor the pulse wave in the brachial artery of the left arm [44, 48]. PPG is usually measured at the body extremities like toes or fingers. In this system, PPG was measured at the level of the arm to retain the fully integrated smart vest design and to avoid using a full sleeved vest or having a long connection between the vest and a separate finger/toe PPG module. The device measured the infrared reflected by the flowing blood volume in the artery. The lag time between R peak from the ECG data and the corresponding pulse wave was used as an estimate for the pulse transit time from the aortic valve to the site where the PPG system is scanning the brachial artery, as shown in Figure 5-12.

When the blood flow pulse travels down to peripheral vasculature, it encounters high flow resistance. So a fraction of the pulse is reflected back and is registered as a (dichrotic) notch within the same pulse waveform. The velocity of the reflected wave varies from individual to individual, and is an indicative of the artery wall stiffness. The lag time for a notch (Δt_{Notch}

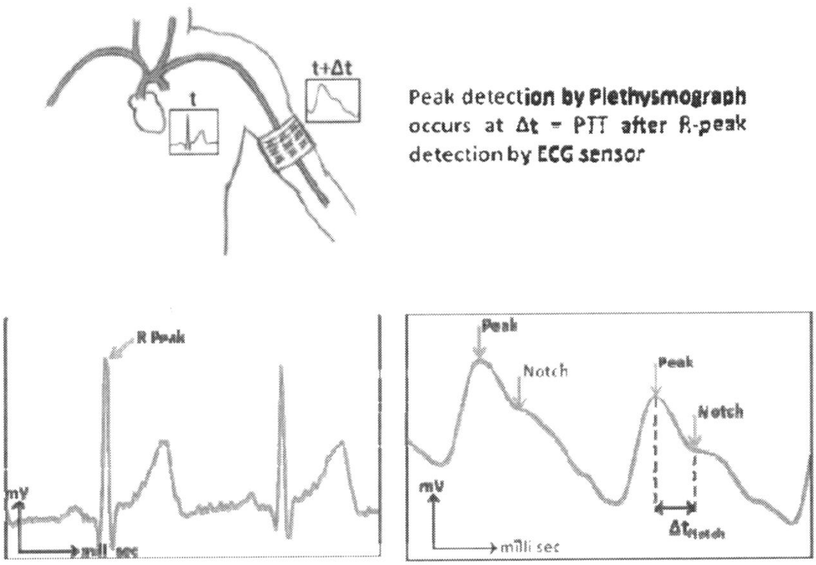

Figure 5-12 Blood pressure measurement system working principle and processing of pulsatile blood flow waveform for blood pressure estimation.

in Figure 5-12) and the height or arm span of the individual can be used as parameters to make an adaptive calibration for pulse transit time based blood pressure estimation.

The blood flow pulse signals from a PPG device and Lead II ECG signals were processed through a peak sorting/filter algorithm for pulse peak and reflected (dichrotic) notch, and R peak time stamp registration respectively. The time stamps were used to determine PTT and Δt_{Notch}. It was found that the error for estimated systolic blood pressure was ±5 mmHg and diastolic blood pressure was ±7 mm Hg. Since a blood pressure variability of ±10 mmHg or higher is considered as medically significant, this system can be applicable to preliminary health monitoring. Since this system provides real time telemedicine data relevant to cardio-vascular system, it can be useful for cardio-vascular healthcare, diagnosis and early detection of a cardiac event. Its connectivity to a cloud server should help in initiating emergency medical responses and prompt communications with medical doctors for e-prescriptions [36].

5.4 Diagnosis of sleep apnea

There are apparent links between deficits in brain chemistry and sleep behavior disorders, such as obstructive sleep apnea (OSA) and rapid eye movement (REM). OSA and REM are common sleep problems that disturb the slumber and daytime behavior of many people. It has been reported that multiple system atrophy, a rare and fatal degenerative neurological disease, is always accompanied by severe sleep disorder. People with OSA show tissue loss in brain regions that help store memory, thus, linking OSA with memory loss and Alzheimer's disease. Obstructive sleep apnea in which breathing temporarily stops during a person's sleep often affects adults but goes undiagnosed in many cases. Its most notable symptoms are snoring and excessive daytime sleepiness, although it can also affect blood pressure, memory, and even reaction time while driving. The sleep disorders are generally undiagnosed and untreated and hundreds of billions of dollars a year are spent due to its related problems on medical costs associated with doctor visits, hospital services, prescriptions, and over-the-counter medications. Moreover, the current sleep lab test systems require a significant facility investment, large instrument capital expenditure, plus the use of many (twenty or more) uncomfortable wired sensors requiring considerable setup labor costs. Thus, there is a need for a low cost, reliable, and ubiquitous patient monitoring system that can be used for sleep monitoring. It is desirable to have a robust and nondisruptive monitoring system that can continuously measure, analyze and record the required parameters while the patient is at home and sleeping in his or her own bed [33].

Sleep apnea is characterized by the repetitive reduction or cessation of breathing during sleep. There are three types of sleep apneas: obstructive sleep apnea (OSA), central sleep apnea (CSA), and mixed sleep apnea. OSA is the most common type of sleep apnea, which is prevalent in 2–4% of adult people, and 20–40% of elderly people. OSA occurs when air cannot be inhaled or exhaled through nasal passages or the mouth, although efforts to breathe continue. CSA is related to brain function. It occurs when the brain fails to send proper signals to the muscles that regulate opening airflow. The cause of mixed sleep apnea is related to both of OSA and CSA. Reduction in blood oxygen saturation and arousal events may occur in all three types of sleep apnea. The blood oxygen level is decreased when the efforts of respiratory muscles are not sufficient to overcome the occlusion. The major symptoms of sleep apnea are drowsiness during the day and snoring. If someone feels fatigued frequently, or awakens with a sensation of gasping or choking suddenly, sleep apnea can be suspected [38]. People with untreated sleep apnea stop breathing repeatedly during their sleep, sometimes hundreds of times during the night and often for one minute or longer. Sleep apnea can cause high blood pressure and other cardiovascular diseases, memory problems, weight gain, impotency, and headaches. Sleep apnea may be responsible for job impairment and motor vehicle accidents. Apart from the physical health risks, sleep apnea can lead to social problems when left undiagnosed or untreated such as a high amount of unnecessary health care cost.

The traditional method for diagnosis of sleep disorder is polysomnography (PSG). PSG is usually performed by a sleep technologist at a sleep center for the full sleep cycle of an individual. PSG records various physiological parameters including EEG, ECG, electromyogram (EMG) of chins and legs, electrooculogram (EOG), nasal airflow, abdominal and thoracic movements, and blood oxygen saturation. PSG is an expensive, inconvenient, and comprehensive method that establishes the manifestation of sleep apnea for an individual patient. Because few centers can afford to perform PSG, this method is not accessible to the general population.

A wireless health monitoring system for diagnosing sleep apnea was proposed, which enables the global monitoring of biomedical signals [38]. A patient does not need hospitalization and can be diagnosed and receive feedback at home. The system supports monitoring five different biomedical signals to diagnose sleep apnea: electrocardiogram with dry electrodes (no gel), body position, nasal airflow, abdomen/chest efforts and oxygen saturation. The system consists of three units: a wireless transmitter, a wireless receiver, and a monitoring unit. The wireless transmitter unit sends the measured signals from sensors to the receiver unit with Zigbee communication. The receiver unit, which has two wireless modules, Zigbee and Wi-Fi, receives signals from the transmitter unit and retransmits signals to the remote monitoring system with Zigbee and Wi-Fi communication, respectively. By using both the Zigbee network and wireless LAN, the system can achieve low power consumption in a local monitoring area with the feature of the Zigbee standard. The system also provides wide data coverage and easily extends its sensor network to the Internet with the Wi-Fi standard. Figure 5-13 shows the data flow for the wireless remote monitoring system.

5.4.1 Sensors

The system supports the measurement of five different biomedical signals, including ECG, body position, nasal airflow, chest effort, and oxygen

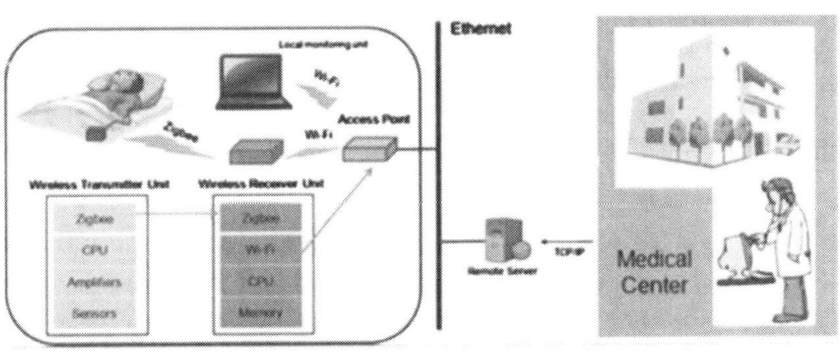

Figure 5-13 Data flow of the wireless health monitoring system network.

saturation. Gold nanowire electrodes, gyroscope, pressure sensor, piezoelectric sensor, and pulse oximeter were utilized to detect the vital signals for the diagnosis of sleep apnea. Figure 5-14 shows the sensors often used in the wireless health monitoring system.

Ag/AgCl and gold electrodes are often used to measure ECG. They require skin preparation to remove dead cells and application of electrolytic gel to reduce the skin contact resistance. However, it is difficult to monitor signals for a long time with gel because of the dry-out of gel and irritation of the skin. The dry-out of gel increased the skin impedance, and results in poor signal quality by inducing noise. These drawbacks can be overcome by using dry nanoelectrodes.

Body position can be recorded with a gyroscope on the body to measure movement patterns during sleep. Nasal airflow can be measured by using a pressure transducer, which can measure the rate of respiration and identify the interruptions in breathing. Abdomen/chest effort or respiration rate is the number of measurement indicative of inspiration and expiration per unit time and it can be measured with piezoelectric or piezoresistive sensors by detecting the movement of abdomen or chest. Oxygen saturation indicates the oxygenation or the amount of oxygen that is being carried in the blood, and it can be measured by a pulse oximeter. An oximeter has

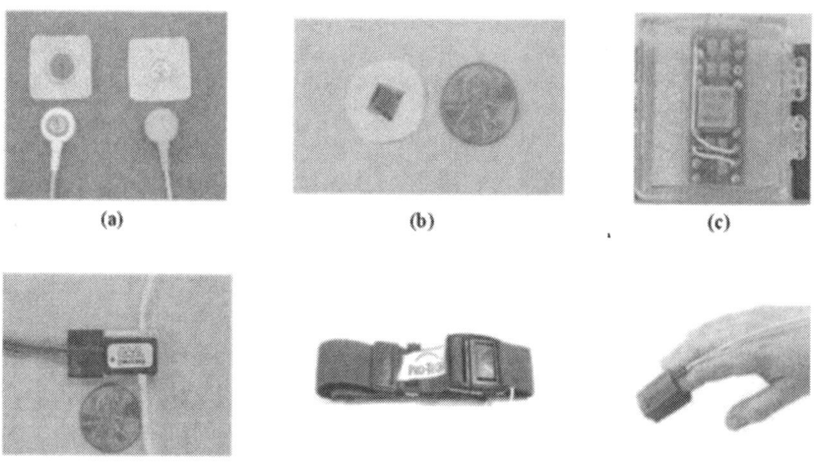

Figure 5-14 Sensors to diagnose sleep apnea: (a) Ag/AgCl skin electrodes for ECG, (b) vertically aligned gold nanowire electrodes for ECG, (c) gyroscope for body position, (d) pressure sensor for nasal airflow, (e) piezoelectric sensor for chest effort, and (f) oximeter for oxygen saturation.

an infrared (IR) /red light-emitting diode (LED) facing a photodiode or a phototransistor. Based on the different absorptions of oxyhemoglobin and deoxyhemoglobin at the wavelengths of IR and red LED, the oxy-/deoxyhemoglobin ratio can be calculated.

5.4.2 Demonstration trial

Demonstration tests were carried out with a wireless remote monitoring system, as shown in figure 5-15. Two gold nanowire electrodes were attached on the right and left upper chest to record Lead I ECG. A belt with a piezoelectric sensor for respiration effort and a gyroscope for body position was placed on the chest. To measure the nasal airflow, nasal prongs were placed in the nostrils. The oximeter was clipped on the finger to measure saturated oxygen level.

Figure 5-16 shows the real-time waveforms of a subject who breathes in normal and abnormal conditions. ECG plot clearly shows the P, QRS, and T waves. The heart rate was obtained by detecting the period of R waves. The amplitude of P wave, QRS complex, T wave, and PR and QT interval durations were also derived to monitor the heart condition, and the results show that all the diagnostic criteria were fulfilled. Body position shows the change of waveform with body movement. The sensitivity of the gyroscope is 25 mV/deg, and the output reveals positive or negative waveforms depending on the rotation direction. Nasal airflow and chest effort were tested under the conditions: absent breathing, normal breathing, and fast breathing. The frequency and amplitude of the waveform were increased in fast breathing

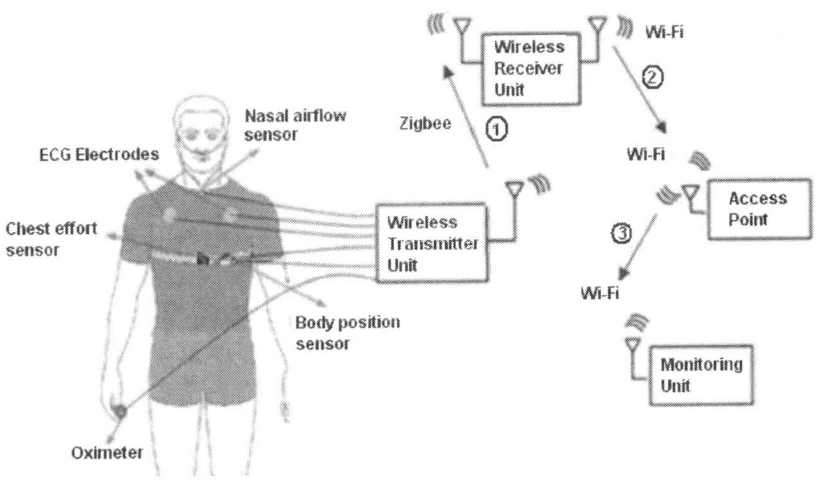

Figure 5-15 Experimental test setup for the wireless remote monitoring system for sleep apnea.

when compared with normal breathing. Because inhaling or exhaling can be identified by the pattern of sensors, negative or positive, the time between inhalation and exhalation can be derived. As the airflow and the chest effort are monitored simultaneously, the case of sleep apnea that has chest effort but does not have airflow can be evaluated. The saturation of peripheral oxygen (S_pO_2) can be derived from the output of the oximeter.

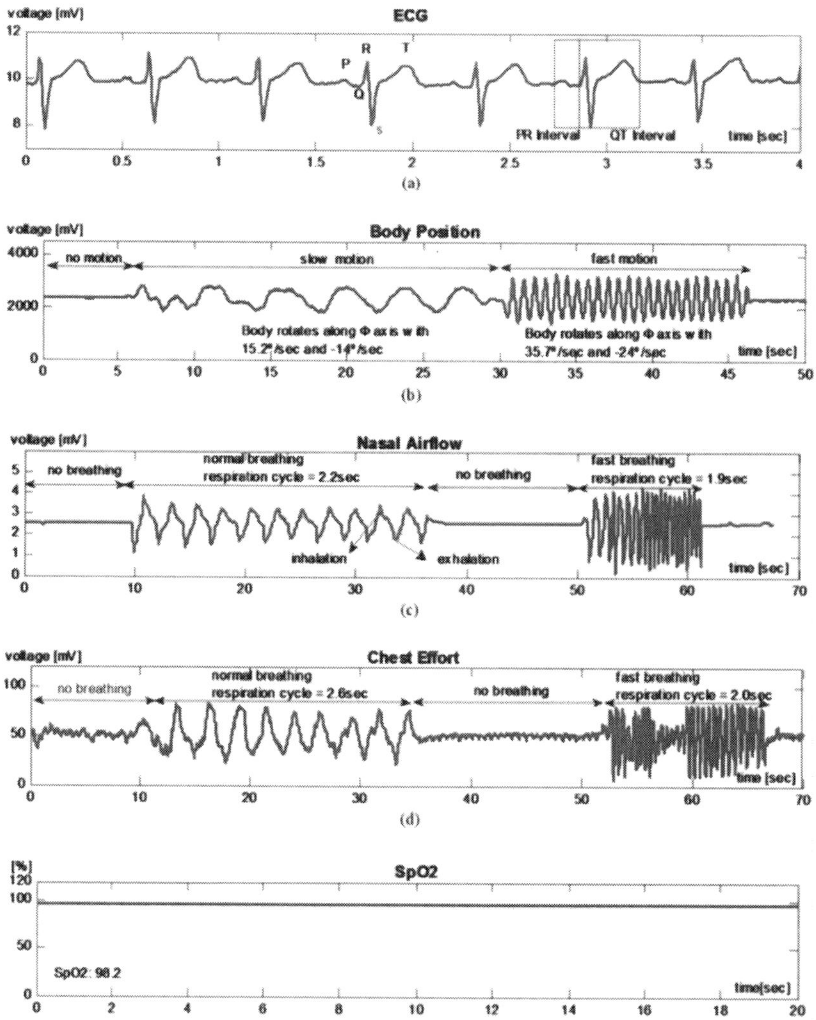

Figure 5-16 Monitored signals: (a) ECG, (b) body position, (c) nasal airflow, (d) chest effort, and (e) oxygen saturation.

6. Perspectives and technical challenges

It is expected that mobile wearable health monitoring systems will transform conventional healthcare practice. However, many technical challenges are hindering progress in the development of mobile wearable health monitoring systems for their practical healthcare applications.

6.1 Transformation of healthcare practice

The conventional health monitoring systems have been limited due to several practical factors, such as lack of wearable and comfortable sensors, lack of wireless standards, and lack of low-power affordable hardware. Due to the latest advances in low-power electronics and wireless protocols, new technologies for long-term and comfortable health monitoring systems have been developed. Smart textiles, coupled with small long-lasting batteries, provide the means to collect data over much longer time scales and in nonclinical settings, and the means for individuals to control the collection and communication of data by easily putting on or taking off the sensors. It can be envisioned that wireless health monitoring will lead to new forms of understanding, diagnosing, and supporting a growing number of individuals [8].

Smartphone-based wireless health monitoring systems offer a convenient solution to the natural progression of healthcare for going mobile [20]. Such systems can be used by healthcare providers to remotely monitor and diagnose the health conditions of patients through Smartphones. Such systems are expected to be popular among healthcare related professions and the public because they are agile, handheld, easy to use and can be used on the move.

The continuous advance of mobile wearable health monitoring systems will potentially transform the future of healthcare [15, 49]. The new health monitoring systems make the clinic visit secondary, placing the communication by mail, text, and voice in first place. In other words, rather than communicating face to face for a few minutes every few weeks or months between a provider and a patient, they can discuss the symptoms and other observations based on the continuous monitoring by mobile wearable health monitoring systems. Further, it has been proven that the capture of vital signs, monitoring of a patient's health data, and remote interaction with the patient can effectively reduce the cost of healthcare while maintaining, and sometimes improving, its quality [50].

6.2 Technical challenges

Before mobile wearable health monitoring systems can be widely accepted by the public and healthcare providers, the following major technical challenges need to be addressed.

6.2.1 Power consumption

Power consumption appears to be the biggest technical issue and performance bottleneck in the development of mobile wearable health monitoring systems [15]. Power management and battery capacity are among the key parameters for the current implementations. For most of the currently available systems, the maximum battery life is about 24 hours, and the power supply takes up about half of the size and weight of the systems.

Besides the improvements in battery technologies [51, 52], implementation of ultra-low power communication electronics, such as Bluetooth version 4.0 standards, will relax the battery capacity requirements. Also, efficient energy optimization methods should be developed. For example, sleep mode method could be used so that the sensor nodes will spend most of their time in a state of low consumption of electricity when data transmission is not required [15].

Many novel methods for energy harvest or conversion are undergoing development [4, 53]. Flexible solar cells and textile coils could be used for supplying energy to mobile wearable health monitoring systems. Energy recovery is also a possible method to reduce the size of the battery. Energy-recovery systems can use, for example, body movement or body heat production, but their efficiency is still quite low at this moment.

6.2.2 Sensors and sensor nodes

Many biosensors used in current health monitoring systems have a bulky size and require very specific on-body placement or body postures to provide reliable measurements. Miniaturization and improvements in sensing mechanisms and fabrication techniques are needed. Also, low-cost, high-efficiency and miniature sensor nodes with wireless capability should be developed to increase the transmission reliability, minimize the interference, and reduce the energy consumption [15, 16]. Nanotechnologies can be used for this purpose [54, 55].

6.2.3 Data security and privacy

Mobile wearable health monitoring systems provide flexible and powerful patient surveillance. However, many patients have privacy concerns about releasing their personal information over open wireless channels. One of the most important issues that healthcare providers must deal with is how to secure the personal information of patients and how to eliminate their privacy concerns [56]. Therefore, proper encryption and authentication mechanisms are required to ensure the privacy of all the communicated data.

6.2.4 Signal noises

Real time acquisitions of physiological signals at the level of skin are susceptible to the noises introduced by the motions of the individual under monitoring. Although a significant reduction of this type of noise is possible by firmly mounting the electrodes on the skin, the requirements for comfort dictate the extent to which the electrodes can be firmly mounted. Besides finding solutions in the hardware, software adaptive digital filters should be developed to remove the residual noises.

6.2.5 Standardization and cooperation

To ensure the interoperability among different communication infrastructures and among different healthcare providers, standardization in communication interfaces and cooperation among different organizations in the development and application of mobile wearable health monitoring systems are needed.

References

1. Hii, P. C., and Chung, W., Y., 2011, "A Comprehensive Ubiquitous Healthcare Solution on an Android™ Mobile Device," *Sensors*, **11**, pp. 6799–6815.
2. Choi, S., Jiang, Z., 2006, "A Novel Wearable Sensor Device with Conductive Fabric and PVDF Film for Monitoring Cardiorespiratory Signals", *Sensors and Actuators A*, **128**, pp. 317–326.
3. Kost, G. J., 1995, "Guidelines for Point-of-Care Testing: Improving Patient Outcomes," *American Journal of Clinical Pathology*, **104**, pp. S111–S127.
4. Axisa, F., Schmitt, P. M., Gehin, C., Delhomme, G., McAdams, E., and Dittmar, A., 2005, "Flexible Technologies and Smart Clothing for Citizen Medicine, Home Healthcare, and Disease Prevention," *IEEE Transactions on Information Technology in Biomedicine*, **9**, pp. 325–336.
5. Monton, E., Hernandez, J. F., Blasco, J. M., Herve, T., Micallef, J., Grech, I., Brincat, A., Traver, V., 2008, "Body Area Network for Wireless Patient Monitoring," *IET Communications*, **2**, pp. 215–222.
6. Shany, T., Redmond, S. J., Narayanan, M. R., and Lovell, N. H., 2012, "Sensors-Based Wearable Systems for Monitoring of Human Movement and Falls," *IEEE Sensors Journal*, **12**, pp. 658–670.
7. Pantelopoulos, A., and Bourbakis, N. G., (2010), "Prognosis - A Wearable Health-Monitoring System for People at Risk: Methodology and Modeling", *IEEE Transactions on Information Technology in Biomedicine*, **14**, pp. 613–621.
8. Fletcher, R. R., Dobson, K., Goodwin, M. S., Eydgahi, H., Wilder-Smith, O., Fernholz, D., Kuboyama, Y., Hedman, E. B., Poh, M. Z., and Picard, R. W., 2010, "iCalm: Wearable Sensor and Network Architecture for Wirelessly Communicating and Logging Autonomic Activity", *IEEE Transactions on Information Technology In Biomedicine*, **14**, pp. 215–223.
9. Yan, L., Bae, J., Lee, S., Roh, T., Song, K., and Yoo, H. J., 2011, "A 3.9 mW 25-Electrode Reconfigured Sensor for Wearable Cardiac Monitoring System", *IEEE Journal of Solid-State Circuits*, **46**, pp. 353–364.
10. Allet, L., Knols, R. H., Shirato K., and de Bruin E. D., 2010, "Wearable Systems for Monitoring Mobility-Related Activities in Chronic Disease: A Systematic Review", *Sensors*, **10**, pp. 9026–9052.
11. Lim, C. K., Luo, Z., Chen, I. M., and Yeo S. H., 2011, "Wearable wireless sensing system for capturing human arm motion", *Sensors and Actuators A*, **166**, pp. 125–132.
12. Gonzalez-Valenzuela, S., Chen, M., and Leung, V. C. M., "Mobility Support for Health Monitoring at Home Using Wearable Sensors", *IEEE Transactions on Information Technology in Biomedicine*, **15**, pp. 539–549.

13. A. Lymberis and D. DeRossi, 2004, *Wearable eHealth Systems for Personalised Health Management.* IOS Press, Amsterdam, The Netherlands.
14. S. Jayaraman, P. Kiekens, and A. Grancaric, 2006, *Intelligent Textiles for Personal Protection and Safety.* IOS Press, Amsterdam, The Netherlands.
15. Pantelopoulos, A., and Bourbakis, N. G., 2010, "A Survey on Wearable Sensor-Based Systems for Health Monitoring and Prognosis", *IEEE Transactions on Systems, Man, and Cybernetics – Part C: Applications and Reviews*, **40**, pp. 1–12.
16. Darwish, A., and Hassanien, A. E., 2011, "Wearable and Implantable Wireless Sensor Network Solutions for Healthcare Monitoring," *Sensors*, **11**, pp. 5561–5595.
17. Egbogah, E. E., and Fapojuwo, A. O., 2011, "A Survey of System Architecture Requirements for Health Care-Based Wireless Sensor Networks," *Sensors*, **11**, pp. 4875–4898.
18. Varadan, V. K., Kumar, P. S., Oh, S., Kwon, H., Rai, P., Banerjee, N., and Harbaugh, R. E., 2011, "e-Nanoflex Sensor System: Smartphone-Based Roaming Health Monitor," *Journal of Nanotechnology in Engineering and Medicine*, **2**, p. 011016.
19. Terry, M., 2010, "Medical apps for smartphones", *Telemedicine and e-Health*, **16**, pp. 17–22.
20. Boulos, M. N. K., Wheeler, S., Tavares, C., and Jones, R., 2011, "How smartphones are changing the face of mobile and participatory healthcare: an overview, with example from eCAALYX," *BioMedical Engineering OnLine*, **10**, p. 24.
21. Park, S., and Jayaraman, S., 2010, "Smart Textile-Based Wearable Biomedical Systems: A Transition Plan for Research to Reality", *IEEE Transactions on Information Technology in Biomedicine*, **14**, pp. 86–92.
22. Zhang, Z. B., Wang, W. D., Shen, Y. H., Wang, B. Q., and J. W., Zheng, 2011, "Design and implementation of Sensing Shirt for Ambulatory Cardiopulmonary Monitoring", *Journal of Medical and Biological Engineering*, **31**, pp. 207–216.
23. Coyle, S., Lau, K. T., Moyna, N., O'Gorman, D., Diamond, D., Di Francesco, F., Costanzo, D., Salvo, P., Trivella, M. G., De Rossi, D. E., Taccini, N., Paradiso, R., Porchet, J. A., Ridolfi, A., Luprano, J., Chuzel, C., Lanier, T., Revol-Cavalier, F., Schoumacker, S., Mourier, V., Chartier, I., Convert, R., De-Moncuit, H., Bini, C., 2010, "BIOTEX-Biosensing Textiles for Personalised Healthcare Management", *IEEE Transactions On Information Technology In Biomedicine*, **14**, pp. 364–370.
24. Goldschlager, N., Goldman, M. J., 1989, *Principle of Clinical Electrocardiography*, 13th Edition, Appleton & Lange, San Mateo, CA.

25. Jahrsdoerfer, M., Giuliano, K., and Dean Stephens, 2005, "Monitoring System Clinical Usefulness of the EASI 12-Lead Continuous Electrocardiographic," *Critical Care Nurse*, **25**, pp. 28–37.
26. Bronzino, J. D., 2006, *Biomedical Engineering Fundamentals*, 2nd ed., CRC, Boca Raton, Florida, pp. (26–2) – (26–3).
27. http://en.wikipedia.org/wiki/Electrocardiography (accessed on May 30, 2012).
28. Tong, S., and Thankor, N. V., 2009, *Quantitative EEG Analysis Methods and Applications*, Artech House, Norwood, MA.
29. Malmivuo, J., and Plonsey, R., 1995, *Bioelectromagnetism*, Chapter 28, Oxford University Press, New York. http://www.bem.fi/book/index.htm (accessed on May 30, 2012).
30. Figueredo, M. V. M., and Dias, J. S., 2004, "Mobile Telemedicine System for Home Care and Patient Monitoring," *Proceedings of the 26th Annual IEEE EMBS International Conference*, **EMBS2004**, pp. 3387–3390.
31. Teplan, M., 2002, "Fundamentals of EEG Measurement," Measurement Science Review, Vol. 2, Institute of Measurement Science, Slovak Academy of Sciences, Bratislava, Slovakia.
32. Zhang, Q., Shi, Y., Teng, D., Dinh, A., Ko, S. B., Chen, L., Basran, J., Dal Bello-Haas, V., and Choi, Y., 2009, "Pulse Transit Time-Based Blood Pressure Estimation Using Hilbert-Huang Transform," *Annual International Conference of the IEEE Engineering in Medicine and Biology Society*, **EMBC 2009**, pp. 1785–1788.
33. V. K., Varadan, Oh, S., Kwon, H., and P., Hankins, 2010, "Wireless Point-of-Care Diagnosis for Sleep Disorder With Dry Nanowire Electrodes," *Journal of Nanotechnology in Engineering and Medicine*, **1**, p. 031012.
34. Kumar, P. S., Oh, S., Rai, P., Kwon, H., Banerjee, N., and Varadan, V. K., 2011, "Design and Implementation of a Bluetooth-Based Band-Aid Pulse Rate Sensor," *Proceedings of SPIE*, **7980**, p. 79800P.
35. Nichols, W. W., O'Rourke, M. F., 1998, *McDonald's Blood Flow in Arteries*, 4th Edition, Oxford University Press, New York, pp. 11–53.
36. Rai, P., Kumar, P. S., Oh, S., Kwon, H., Mathur, G. N., Varadan, V. K., and Agarwal, M. P., 2012, "Smart healthcare textile sensor system for unhindered-pervasive health monitoring," *Proceedings of SPIE*, **8344**, p. 83440E.
37. Kim, J., Yang, S. Y., Lee, M. H., Kim, J. H.; Cai, Z., Kim, J. H., Kang, K. S., 2008, "Cellulose smart material for sensor, actuator and MEMS applications.", *Proceedings of the ASME Conference on Smart Materials, Adaptive Structures and Intelligent Systems*, **1**, pp. 31–32.
38. Oh, S., Kwon, H., and V. K., Varadan, 2011, "Ubiquitous Health Monitoring System for Diagnosis of Sleep Apnea With Zigbee Network

and Wireless LAN," *Journal of Nanotechnology in Engineering and Medicine*, **2**, p. 021008.

39. Free, C., Phillips, G., Felix, L., Galli, L., Patel, V., Edwards P., 2010, "The Effectiveness of M-Health Technologies for Improving Health and Health Services: A Systematic Review Protocol," *BMC Research Notes*, **3**, p. 250.
40. Varadan, V. K., Kumar, P. S., Oh, S., Kegley, L., and P., Rai, 2011, "e-bra With Nanosensors for Real Time Cardiac Health Monitoring and Smartphone Communication," *Journal of Nanotechnology in Engineering and Medicine*, **2**, p. 021011.
41. Kailanto, H., Hyvarinen, E., Hyttinen, J., 2008, "Mobile ECG Measurement and Analysis System Using Mobile Phone as the Base Station," *Second International Conference on Pervasive Computing Technologies for Healthcare*, pp. 12–14.
42. Rai, P., Kumar, P. S., Oh, S., Kwon, H., Mathur, G. N., and Varadan, V. K., 2011, "Printable Low-Cost Sensor Systems for Healthcare Smart Textiles," *Proceedings of SPIE*, **7980**, p. 79800E.
43. Pan, J., Tompkins, W. J., 1985, "A Real-Time QRS Detection Algorithm," *IEEE Transactions on Biomedical Engineering*, **32**, pp. 230–236.
44. Laurent, C., Jonsson, B., Vegfors, M., Lindberg, L., G., 2005, "Non-Invasive Measurement of Systolic Blood Pressure on the Arm Utilising Photoplethysmography: Development of the Methodology," *Medical & Biological Engineering & Computing*, **43**, pp. 131–135.
45. Lodha, R., Mukerji, N., Sinha, N., Pandey, R., M., and Jain, Y., "Is Axillary Temperature an Appropriate Surrogate for Core Temperature?" *Indian Journal of Pediatrics*, **67** (8), pp. 571–574. (2000).
46. Task Force of the European Society of Cardiology the North American Society of Pacing Electrophysiology, 1996, "Heart Rate Variability: Standards of Measurement, Physiological Interpretation, and Clinical Use", *Circulation*, **93**, pp. 1043–1065.
47. Khoor, S., Nieberl, J., Fugedi, K., Kail, E., 2001, "Telemedicine ECG-Telemetry with Bluetooth Technology," *Computer in Cardiology*, **28**, pp. 585–588.
48. Allen, J., 2007, "Photoplethysmography and Its Application in Clinical Physiological Measurement," *Physiological Measurement*, **28**, pp. R1–R39.
49. Waegemann, C. P., 2010, "mHealth: The Next Generation of Telemedicine?" *Telemedicine and e-Health*, **16**, pp. 23–25.
50. Noel, H. C., Vogel, D. C., Erdos, J. J., Cornwall, D., Levin, F., 2004, "Home Telehealth Reduces Healthcare Costs", *Telemedicine Journal and e-Health*, **10**, pp. 170–183.
51. Chiang, Y. M., 2010, "Building a Better Battery", *Science*, **330**, pp. 1485–1486.
52. Kang, B., and Ceder, G., 2009, "Battery Materials for Ultrafast Charging and Discharging", *Nature*, **458**, pp. 190–193.

53. Yan, L., Yoo, J., Kim, B., and Yoo, H. J., 2010, "A 0.5-μV_{rms} 12-μW Wirelessly Powered Patch-Type Healthcare Sensor for Wearable Body Sensor Network", *IEEE Journal of Solid-State Circuits*, **45**, pp. 2356–2365.
54. Varadan, V. K., Chen, L. F., and Xie, J., 2008, *Nanomedicine: Design and Applications of Magnetic Nanomaterials, Nanosensors and Nanosystems*, John Wiley & Sons, Ltd., Chichester, West Sussex, UK.
55. Tolani, S. B., Craig, M., DeLong, R. K., Ghosh, K, Wanekaya, A. K., 2009, "Towards Biosensors Based on Conducting Polymer Nanowires", *Analytical and Bioanalytical Chemistry*, **393**, pp. 1225–1231.
56. Ren, Y., Pazzi, R. W. N., and Boukerche, A., 2010, "Monitoring Patients via a Secure and Mobile Healthcare System", *IEEE Wireless Communications*, **17**, pp. 59–65.

CPSIA information can be obtained at www.ICGtesting.com
Printed in the USA
BVOW062251150713

325738BV00004BA/21/P